3018
WM 896.

Down Syndrome and Alzheimer's Disease

Biological correlates

Edited by
Vee P Prasher

Consultant Neuro-Psychiatrist
South Birmingham Primary Care Trust
and
Honorary Senior Research Fellow
King's College London

Foreword by
Trevor Parmenter

D1419733

Radcliffe Publishing
Oxford • Seattle

Radcliffe Publishing Ltd
18 Marcham Road
Abingdon
Oxon OX14 1AA
United Kingdom

www.radcliffe-oxford.com
Electronic catalogue and worldwide online ordering facility.

British Library Cataloguing in Publication Data

A catalogue record for this book is available from the British Library.

ISBN-10 1 85775 637 1
ISBN-13 978 1 85775 637 1

Typeset by Anne Joshua & Associates, Oxford
Printed and bound by TJ International Ltd, Padstow, Cornwall

To Dr Vallepur HR Krishnan, Consultant in Developmental Psychiatry,
Little Plumstead Hospital, Norwich, Norfolk

Contents

Foreword

In the century 1850–1950 scientific inquiry into intellectual disability was essentially characterised by a focus on the physical characteristics of people with this diagnosis, including those with Down syndrome. In 1866 Langdon Down, after whom the syndrome was named, reported that the physical features of many of his patients at London Hospital and the Earlwood Asylum resembled the Mongolian race. He also pointed out that the condition appeared to cross racial boundaries. Concerning possible aetiology, he suggested that it was inherited from tuberculosis in the parents. It was not until 1959 that Lejeune and colleagues made the discovery that the extra chromosome was the underlying cause of Down syndrome.

In general terms, the last half of the twentieth century witnessed a major shift away from the "medical" model of disability which had sought to describe, diagnose, classify and treat impairments; to an emphasis upon the "social" model that grew out of a combination of philosophical, advocacy and human rights movements. Many condemned the medical model for its supposed pessimism about the educability of people with an intellectual disability, but significantly Langdon Down reported on the positive effects of training as did Seguin before him.

The "schism" between the medical and social models to some extent became evident in the world congresses of the International Association for the Scientific Study of Intellectual Disabilities (IASSID) where there was a polarisation of two distinctive themes; one exploring traditional medical aspects and the other concentrating upon community living and social aspects of the lives of people with an intellectual disability. The emergence of Special Interest Research Groups (SIRGs) in the 1990s, spearheaded by the Ageing SIRG, has significantly helped to integrate the medical and social aspects of scientific inquiry. The issue of the early onset of dementia in adults with an intellectual disability, especially those with Down syndrome, has been a special focus of the work of this group.

The publication of this book, which brings together in one volume major biological aspects concerning dementia in Alzheimer's disease (DAD) in adults with Down syndrome, is particularly significant for at least three reasons. First, the very biological bases underpinning the development of dementia in Alzheimer's disease provide an important bridge between basic research in the general population and that in the area of Down syndrome and in intellectual disability generally. This provides an excellent opportunity for a cross fertilisation of efforts. Not only is dementia in Alzheimer's disease emerging as the greatest challenge for those charged with the health and community care of people who are ageing with an intellectual disability; it is a similar challenge for the dramatically increasing numbers of older people in the general population. It is somewhat ironic that whilst better healthcare and improved life style (at least in the developed world) has lengthened life expectancy for all, society is being challenged by the possibility of the increased exposure of the ageing population to disease and disability.

Second, it provides a comprehensive "state of the art" analysis of the biological correlates of DAD and Down syndrome from a variety of scientific perspectives including genetics, biochemistry, neurophysiology, neuropathology, neuropsychiatry and neuroimaging.

Third, this analysis also provides a clear indication as to where future research efforts need to be targeted, especially in the development of reliable markers that might improve clinical diagnostic accuracy and assist early detection. Presently the clinical diagnosis of DAD is fraught with imprecision and, even when accurate, may be made at the end of a long process of hidden neuropathology.

The scientific community investigating one of the most serious health challenges facing adults with an intellectual disability is indebted to Dr Vee Prasher and colleagues for this scholarly contribution to the study of the biological correlates of dementia in Alzheimer's disease in adults with Down syndrome. This important collection of the most recent research findings in this field of enquiry will further stimulate efforts to develop treatments that may ameliorate the condition; delay its onset, and ultimately provide means for prevention.

Trevor R. Parmenter AMPhD FACE FAAMR FIASSID FASSID
Past President of IASSID (1996–2000)
University of Sydney
May 2006

Preface

To fully appreciate the recent advances in the clinical and cognitive aspects of dementia in Alzheimer's disease (DAD) in adults with Down syndrome, an awareness of the essential biological aspects underlying the disease process is essential. Furthermore, in view of a number of significant developments in our knowledge of basic brain mechanisms and in aspects of neuroscience affecting Alzheimer's disease in the general population, it is important that a resource is made available which critically appraises the important biological aspects of DAD in older adults with Down syndrome. This book aims to provide for researchers and clinicians in the field of intellectual disability a resource on recent neuro-psychiatric developments in Alzheimer's disease which may supplement existing clinical knowledge.

This book endeavours to bring together in one place recent research findings relating to the neuropathology, genetics, blood markers and neurophysiological aspects of Alzheimer's disease in older adults with Down syndrome. To date, the majority of interest in this area has been focused on the clinical and diagnostic aspects of DAD in the intellectually disabled population. Until recently the underlying biological abnormalities, which possibly give rise to the clinical psychopathology of DAD in individuals with Down syndrome, have been neglected. To our knowledge this book is the first in the field of intellectual disability to have been published in order to address this concern.

The overall goal of this book is to help researchers and clinicians working with people with intellectual disability to better understand the biomedical abnormalities of DAD, and to facilitate interest and further research into the fundamentals of Alzheimer's disease in adults with Down syndrome.

A few comments are needed on the terminology adopted in this text. The term 'Alzheimer's disease' has been used to denote the neuropathological disease process, while 'dementia in Alzheimer's disease' has been used to refer to the clinical aspects of the neurodegenerative condition. It is accepted that such terms have not yet gained universal acceptance. In addition, the term 'intellectual disabilities' is used to denote what the International Association for the Scientific Study of Intellectual Disabilities (IASSID) refers to as intellectual disability. This term is used synonymously with 'mental retardation', 'learning disabilities', 'mental handicap' and 'intellectual handicap.'

Vee P Prasher
May 2006
vprasher@compuserve.com

About the editor

Vee P Prasher is a Consultant Psychiatrist in Neurodevelopmental Psychiatry in Birmingham and a Senior Research Fellow at King's College London. He graduated from Birmingham University in 1985 and has subsequently completed MMedSci, MD and PhD postgraduate degrees. His main research interests are ageing and the physical health of adults with Down syndrome. He has published over 100 research articles and edited or written a number of textbooks on intellectual disabilities. In 2004 he was conferred the title of Fellow of the International Association for the Scientific Study of Intellectual Disabilities.

List of contributors

Felix Beacher BA, MSc
Researcher
Institute of Psychiatry
London, UK

Mark J Dickinson BSc, MBBS, MRCPsych
Consultant Psychiatrist in Learning Disability
Chase Farm Hospital
Middlesex, UK

Satnam Kunar MBChB MRCPsych
Researcher
Greenfields
Monyhull
Birmingham, UK

David M A Mann PhD, FRCPath
Professor of Neuropathology
University of Manchester
Manchester, UK

Pankaj D Mehta PhD
Research Scientist and Head of Department of Humoral
Immunology
New York Institute for Basic Research in Developmental Disabilities
New York, USA

Declan G M Murphy PhD, FRCPsych
Professor of Psychiatry and Brain Maturation
Institute of Psychiatry
London, UK

Robert J Pary MD
Professor of Psychiatry
Southern Illinois University School of Medicine
Springfield
Illinois, USA

Maire Percy PhD
Director, Neurogenetics Laboratory
Surrey Place Centre
Professor of Physiology (Emeritus) and Obstetrics and Gynaecology
University of Toronto
Toronto, Canada

Vee P Prasher MD, PhD, MRCPsych
Consultant Neuropsychiatrist
Greenfields
Monyhull
Birmingham
and
Honorary Senior Research Fellow
King's College London
London, UK

Gautam Rajendran MBBS
Child Psychiatry Fellow
University of Colorado Health Sciences Center
Denver
Colorado, USA

Nicole Schupf PhD
Associate Professor of Clinical Epidemiology
Taub Institute for Research on Alzheimer's Disease and the Aging Brain
Columbia University Medical Center
New York, USA

Iqbal Singh
Consultant Psychiatrist
Hillingdon Hospital
Uxbridge
Middlesex
and
Honorary Senior Clinical Lecturer
Imperial School of Medicine
London, UK

Andrea Stonecipher MD
Psychiatry Resident
Southern Illinois University School of Medicine
Springfields
Illinois, USA

Frank E Visser MD, PhD
Consultant Neurophysiologist
's Heeren Loo Midden Nederland Ermelo
The Netherlands

List of abbreviations

Aβ	amyloid β-peptide
ABS	adaptive behavior scale
AChE	acetylcholinesterase
ACT	α-1-antichymotrypsin
ACTH	adrenocorticotropic hormone
AD	Alzheimer's disease
AEP	auditory evoked potential
ApoE	apolipoprotein E
APP	amyloid precursor protein
BACE	beta-site amyloid precursor protein-cleaving enzyme
CAMDEX	Cambridge Examination for Mental Disorders of the Elderly
ChAT	choline acetyltransferase
CRH	corticotrophin-releasing hormone
Cr+PCr	creatine and phosphocreatine
CSF	cerebrospinal fluid
CT	computerised tomography
DAD	dementia in Alzheimer's disease
DMR	Dementia Questionnaire for Mentally Retarded Persons
DS	Down syndrome
DSDS	Dementia Scale for Down Syndrome
DSM–III	*Diagnostic and Statistical Manual of Mental Disorders – Third Edition*
DSM–IV	*Diagnostic and Statistical Manual of Mental Disorders – Fourth Edition*
ECF	extracellular fluid
EEG	electroencephalography
ELISA	enzyme-linked immunosorbent assay
FAD	familial form of Alzheimer's disease
HDL	high-density lipoprotein
^{1}H-MRS	proton magnetic resonance spectroscopy
HPT	hypothalamic–pituitary–thyroid axis
HSPG	heparan sulphate proteoglycan
ICD–9	*International Classification of Diseases and Related Health Problems – Ninth Revision*
ICD–10	*International Classification of Diseases and Related Health Problems – Tenth Revision*
ID	intellectual disability
LDL	low-density lipoprotein
LOMEDS	late-onset myoclonic epilepsy in adults with Down syndrome
MCI	mild cognitive impairment
MCV	mean corpuscular volume
MDT	multi-disciplinary team
MMSE	Mini Mental State Examination
MRI	magnetic resonance imaging

NAA	*N*-acetylaspartate
NFT	neurofibrillary tangles
NSF	National Service Framework
PET	positron emission tomography
PHF	paired helical filaments
PS1	presenilin 1
PS2	presenilin 2
rCBF	regional cerebral blood flow
SIB–R	Scale of Independent Behaviour – Revised
SOD1	superoxide dismutase-1
SP	senile plaques
SPECT	single photon emission computed tomography
T3	triiodothyronine
T4	thyroxine
TBG	thyroxine-binding globulin
TBP	thyroxine-binding proteins
Tg	thyroglobulin
TRH	thyroid-releasing hormone
TSH	thyroid-stimulating hormone
VBM	voxel-based morphometry
VEP	visual evoked potential
VLDL	very-low-density lipoprotein

Chapter 1

Overview of Alzheimer's disease in Down syndrome

Robert J Pary, Gautam Rajendran and Andrea Stonecipher

Introduction

It may seem strange, but there is good news about people with Down syndrome (DS) being at risk for Alzheimer's disease (AD). A century ago, babies with DS seldom lived long enough to develop AD! In the early twentieth century the average lifespan of a child with DS was 9 years.[1] Just over two decades ago, the median age of death for people with DS was 25 years.[2] At the start of the new millennium the average life expectancy is now only 15–20 years less than that for the general population.

In contrast to the many books and articles written by and for parents about the experience of raising a child with DS, very little has been written about the personal experience of families in dealing with a family member who has both DS and dementia in Alzheimer's disease (DAD). It was not until the last decade of the twentieth century that texts written specifically for parents of people with DS began to include the issue of dementia.[3] Family accounts are now being published. Margaret T Fray has written about the challenging experience of caring for her sister with DS and dementia.[4] Unfortunately, Fray's book is not readily accessible in many countries.

As a result of medical advances, it is now common for a person with DS to live to over 60 years of age.[5] In contrast to the general population, men with DS live longer than women with DS. In 2000, the median life expectancy was 61.1 years for men and 57.8 years for women.[6] Furthermore, not everyone with DS develops DAD, although the risk is considerable. Some service planners are beginning to believe that the actual numbers of people with DS and DAD may be lower than was previously thought, although they are still quite substantial.[7] Approximately 50–60% of adults with DS will develop DAD by the age of 60 to 70 years.[8] However, there are case reports in the literature of elderly individuals with DS but without DAD.

Chicoine and McGuire[9] describe the case of 'Ann', an 83-year-old woman with DS. On physical examination, she had several characteristic features of DS, including a flattened occiput, eyelids that slanted upward, prominent epicanthal folds, Brushfield spots (mottled or speckled areas on the iris), small palate, bilateral valgus-curving of the fifth finger, small hands and small feet. Furthermore, she had health problems commonly associated with DS, including bilateral hallux valgus, bilateral cataracts, and dystrophic toenails with onychomycosis. Chromosome analysis revealed mosaic 21 (75% had trisomy 21 and 25% were normal). 'Ann' died one month after suffering a hip fracture. Prior to death she had not shown signs of dementia, such as loss of memory or loss of skills (except those explained by the hip fracture).

However, whatever 'positive spin' one gives the increased risk of AD in individuals with DS soon disappears when the reality of DAD hits, as it did in the case of Margaret T Fray's sister.[4] Alzheimer's disease robs a person of his or her connection to loved ones and eventually to him- or herself.

History of dementia and Down syndrome

Functional deterioration in adults with DS has been noted since the nineteenth century. In 1876, Fraser and Mitchel[10] wrote that individuals with DS had a 'sort of precipitated senility.' As was mentioned above, a century ago few children with DS survived to teenage years. It is therefore somewhat surprising that post-mortem evidence of AD in an adult with DS was described as early as 1929[11] according to Lott.[12] In the mid-twentieth century, Jervis was the first clinician to suggest that AD complicates ageing in older adults with DS.[13]

One of the seminal observations of recent history has been the detection of AD neuropathology (senile plaques and neurofibrillary tangles) in the brains of adults with DS who are older than 35 years.[14] The belief in the inevitability of AD changes in the post-mortem brains of adults with DS significantly affected the way in which clinicians, carers and family members approached the ageing process of older adults with DS in the 1980s and 1990s. Furthermore, prevalence studies became extremely important, and will be discussed in detail. The neuropathology of AD in people with DS will be discussed in Chapter 2 of this book.

Epidemiology of dementia in individuals with Down syndrome

Accurate information about the prevalence (i.e. the total number of cases) of DAD in DS is critical if erroneous clinical attitudes are to be avoided. A 1994 international conference concluded that 'estimates of overall and age-specific rates of Alzheimer-type dementia in adults with DS . . . vary widely (from under 10% to over 75%).'[15] However, an article published within the past decade still referred to the inevitability of DAD in individuals over 40 years of age with DS. Martin[16] advised that 'early AD occurs in almost 100% of DS patients over 40 years old.' Smith[17] argued forcefully against this pessimistic view in a Letter-to-the-Editor response to Martin's article. Martin did recommend ruling out reversible causes first. However, clinicians who believe in the inevitability of DAD in people over 40 years of age with DS will probably fail to search aggressively for potential reversible causes of the decline.

There are several methodological challenges in accurately determining the epidemiology of dementia in individuals with DS. One fundamental difficulty is that some studies use phenotypic rather cytogenetic diagnosis of DS.[18] The problem with using phenotypic criteria alone for the diagnosis of DS has been highlighted previously,[19] and became apparent to one of the authors (RJP) during a psychiatric consultation. The individual concerned was 45 years old and had been diagnosed with DS during infancy by her family doctor. She had short stature, intellectual disability (ID) and an upward slant to her eyes (she was of Asian descent). However, she did not have a palmar crease, Brushfield spots, flattened occiput, valgus-angled fifth finger or a space between her first and second toes. What was most suspicious of all was that she looked at least ten years younger than her chronological age. Her middle-class, college-educated family never questioned the diagnosis of DS, and karotyping was never undertaken. Although the individual had several behavioural challenges, none of them would lead one to suspect dementia or a behavioural phenotype of DS.

Although lack of chromosomal confirmation can be problematic in large population surveys, there are other potential limitations. Bush and Beail[20] discussed several other methodological issues in accurately determining the prevalence of dementia in people with DS, including cohort bias in cross-sectional designs, the lack of a standardised protocol to rule out potentially reversible causes of functional decline, non-standardised diagnostic criteria and inadequate evaluations of premorbid cognitive functioning. Cohort bias in cross-sectional designs refers to two potential problems. One is the problem of conducting prevalence studies exclusively using subjects living in an institution. The lack of educational, cultural or vocational stimulation in an institution can result in individuals appearing regressed.[21] Similarly, the shock of being admitted to an institution, especially if someone has lived all of one's life prior to this at home, could cause a temporary regression in functioning. A cross-sectional study would only report a decline. In addition, as Bush and Beail[20] emphasise, some individuals may be admitted to an institution while in the very early stages of dementia. All of these factors can result in overestimation of the prevalence rates of DAD in adults with DS living in an institution. If individuals with DS in a longitudinal study die from non-dementia-related causes, the surviving cohort may be skewed.[20] This means that as members of the cohort group die, but never developed dementia, the percentage (and significance) of those survivors who do develop dementia may be unduly increased.

Another major issue in some studies has been the lack of a standardised protocol to eliminate other causes of functional decline. The differential diagnosis of dementia in DS will be covered in detail later. Bush and Beail[20] point out that some early researchers assumed that any functional decline in older adults with DS had to be due to AD. Cross-sectional studies would be at increased risk for this kind of error.

A third major problem is the use of non-standardised diagnostic criteria for dementia in individuals with DS.[20] Some researchers will estimate different odds ratios of dementia according to how stringently the diagnostic criteria for dementia are defined. Zigman and colleagues studied 2534 people with DS and 16 182 people with ID due to other causes,[18] and found significantly different rates depending on the strictness of the criteria for dementia.

One solution to the lack of standardised diagnostic criteria has been the formation of an international Working Group for the Establishment of Criteria for the Diagnosis of Dementia in Individuals with Intellectual Disability.[22] This working group endorsed a test battery that included a number of different scales. Some tests which could be used as part of the test battery include (i) the Dementia Questionnaire for Mentally Retarded Persons (DMR),[23] (ii) the Dementia Scale for Down Syndrome (DSDS),[24] (iii) the Reiss Screen[25] Scale of Independent

Behaviour–Revised (SIB–R)[26] and (iv) the Adaptive Behaviour Scale.[27] These scales were just the ones administered to informants. In addition, there were 11 other scales to be administered to the individual! Unfortunately, the battery is too unwieldy for clinical work (as well as for most research studies). The proposed test battery is a worthy preliminary endeavour, but is in need of 'pruning' before it can be widely used in the field.

A recent multi-centre evaluation of screening tools for dementia in older adults with ID (including 26 out of 38 individuals with DS) did not use the working group's complete test battery (although it did use parts of it).[28] Schultz and colleagues[28] concluded that there is still not a 'gold standard', although they found both the DSDS[24] and the DMR[23] useful.

With the above-mentioned cautions, the following are several representative prevalence studies of DS and AD. Lai[29] describes findings representative of prevalence studies in institutionalised individuals with DS. Lai's group followed 53 individuals with DS over the age of 35 years, and found that 6% had dementia in the 35–49 years age cohort, 55% in the 50–59 years cohort and 100% in the cohort aged 60 years or over (an earlier report from the group had estimated the prevalence in people over 60 years of age to be 75%).

In contrast, a study by Sekijima and colleagues of institutionalised adults with DS in Japan found a lower prevalence.[30] They described 106 individuals who were 30 years or older. The number of individuals who were diagnosed clinically with DS compared with the number for whom confirmation was obtained with chromosomal analysis was not given. None of the 39 individuals aged 30 to 39 years had dementia. Among those aged 40 to 49 years, 7 out of 43 (16%) had dementia, and among those aged 50 to 59 years, 9 out of 22 (41%) had dementia. Neither of the two individuals aged over 60 years had dementia.

Visser and colleagues[31] followed 307 patients with DS who were monitored for 5 to 10 years prospectively in order to determine the prevalence of DAD in an institutionalised setting. Clinical signs, cognitive functioning and electroencephalograms were assessed. Whenever possible, post-mortem neuropathological examinations were performed. Progressive mental and physical deterioration was found in 56 of the institutionalised patients. The mean age at onset of dementia was 56 years. The prevalence increased from 11% between the ages of 40 and 49 years to 77% between the ages of 60 and 69 years, and all patients over 70 years of age had dementia. Visser's group[31] reported that the neuropathological findings were consistent with the clinical diagnosis.

Future prevalence studies will not only need to include chromosomal analysis of all of the participants, but will also need to determine whether the karyotype was atypical. Some reports are already providing numbers of atypical karyotypes.[32] Schupf[33] notes mosaicism in both 'Ann', the 83-year-old woman with DS described by Chicoine and McGuire,[9] and a 74-year-old woman without dementia. 'Ann' had 25% disomy for chromosome 21, and the 74-year-old woman without signs of DAD had 86% disomy. Schupf[33] believes that atypical karyotypes, such as translocations, partial trisomies and mosaicism, may have a lower risk for AD.

Introduction to the genetics of Alzheimer's disease and Down syndrome

The increased risk of AD in DS is attributed to a gene found on chromosome 21, for *amyloid precursor protein (APP)*, although the trigger for development of dementia is unknown.[33] APP has three copies in DS because of trisomy 21. Amyloid is accumulated extracellularly in senile plaques, a characteristic feature of the neuropathology of AD. APP is cleaved by proteases, β- and γ-secretase.[34] A product of APP is the amyloid β-peptide, Aβ1–42, which is selectively increased in early-onset familial AD.[34] Amyloid β-peptide can be measured in the plasma. Schupf and colleagues[35] noted that levels of the amyloid peptides Aβ1–42 and Aβ1–40 were higher in adults with DS than in controls. In the general population, elevated plasma Aβ1–42 levels may indicate an increased risk of AD.[36] (For further details on the association between amyloid and AD in DS, *see* Chapters 3 and 4.) Another gene of interest on chromosome 21 is that for superoxide dismutase-1 (SOD1).[37] SOD1 consists of 154 amino acids and is involved in oxygen metabolism.[38] (For further information on SOD1 and AD in DS, *see* Chapter 5.)

Although it does not occur on chromosome 21, an apolipoprotein E (ApoE) genotype is associated with AD.[39] ApoE appears to be involved in the transportation of cholesterol. There are three alleles, namely ϵ2, ϵ3 and ϵ4. Research investigating ApoE and AD in individuals with DS has not yielded consistent findings, but according to Schupf[33] the ApoE ϵ4 allele appears to be associated with an earlier onset of dementia. In contrast, ApoE ϵ2 offers some protection and is associated with a reduced risk of dementia. This topic is covered in detail in Chapter 3.

Natural history of dementia in individuals with Down syndrome

A study by Thase and colleagues[40] was one of the first to note a significant increase in apathy in institutionalised individuals with DS aged 50 years or older ($n = 29$) compared with control groups ($n = 24$). Interestingly, individuals with DS aged 31 to 40 years had significantly lower apathy scores than controls. Although Thase and colleagues[40] did not formally diagnose dementia, they found significantly lower scores for orientation, digit span, visual memory, object naming and general knowledge in individuals with DS compared with controls.

Evenhuis[41] described the natural history of dementia in DS. She followed 17 middle-aged patients with DS until death. In total, 14 individuals had a clinical diagnosis of dementia and autopsy features of Alzheimer-like changes. The clinical pattern of deterioration was different in individuals with moderate ID compared with those with severe ID, although the numbers were small (9 *vs.* 5). In individuals with moderate ID and DS, early symptoms of dementia recognised by the staff included apathy, withdrawal, daytime sleepiness and loss of self-help skills.[41] Interestingly, memory disturbance was part of the early presentation in only three out of nine individuals. It was not until the second or third year that symptoms of remote memory loss, disorientation and apraxia (loss of ability to perform tasks despite intact motor and sensory functioning) were detectable. Also by the third year the remaining six individuals with moderate ID showed recent memory loss.

Evenhuis[41] reported that, in contrast to individuals with both DS and moderate ID, adults with severe ID and DS showed apathy, loss of self-help skills, loss of gait and seizures during the first year of dementia. Evenhuis[41] could not demonstrate cognitive deterioration in individuals with severe ID. In support of Evenhuis' observation of increased seizures and dementia, a study published by Van Buggenhout and colleagues[42] found that 9 out of 18 individuals with dementia had seizures. Furthermore, Van Buggenhout's group believed that the onset of seizures was often one of the first signs of DAD if it occurred in older adults with DS.

Lai[29] also described a different pattern of deterioration depending upon whether the person with DS had higher functioning or more severe ID. Memory impairment, temporal disorientation and reduced verbal output were the initial findings in higher-functioning adults with DS. In contrast, those individuals with more severe ID became less interactive with others and this was the initial hallmark of dementia. The second phase showed a decline in activities of daily living, slowed gait and the emergence of seizures. Seizures usually developed within two years of the onset of dementia. In the final phase, individuals became bedridden and incontinent.[29]

Like Evenhuis,[41] Holland and colleagues[43] found that the early deterioration was more often in personality and behaviour than in memory. These researchers used a modified version of the Cambridge Examination for Mental Disorders of the Elderly (CAMDEX)[44] to diagnose dementia. Holland and colleagues found that 10 out of 18 individuals (55%) showed apathy, while only 2 out of 18 (11%) experienced memory loss as the first change.[43] Loss of self-help skills occurred in only 3 out of 18 individuals (17%). The authors of the study believed that frontal lobe deficits were manifested early because of reduced cerebral capacity in individuals with DS.

In the general population, apathy is considered by some to be the most common behaviour resulting from AD.[45] The frontal subcortical circuitry appears to be involved. The study of apathy is plagued by imprecise definitions. Landes and colleagues[45] emphasise that some researchers have defined apathy as an absence of emotion or as emotional withdrawal. They note that others also include lowered initiative, reduced physical activities, indifference to activities, decreased responsiveness, poor persistence and fatigue. The distinction between apathy and depression will be discussed in the section on differential diagnosis.

In contrast to Evenhuis[41] and Holland,[43] Oliver and colleagues[46] focused mainly on cognitive change. They conducted a four-year prospective study of age-related cognitive change in adults with DS, which revealed that although neuropathological studies indicate a high risk for DAD in adults with DS, neuropsychological studies suggest a lower prevalence of dementia. In this study, cognitive deterioration in adults ($n = 57$) with DS was examined prospectively over a period of four years in order to establish the rates and profiles of cognitive deterioration. Assessments of domains of cognitive function that are known to change with the onset of dementia were employed. These included tests of learning, memory, orientation, agnosia, apraxia and aphasia, and the individual growth trajectory methodology was used to analyse change over time. Severe cognitive deterioration, such as acquired apraxia and agnosia, was evident in 28% of individuals aged over 30 years, and a higher prevalence of these impairments was associated with older age. The rate of cognitive deterioration also increased with age and degree of pre-existing cognitive impairment. In addition, deterioration in memory, learning and orientation preceded the acquisition of aphasia, agnosia and apraxia, which suggests that the prevalence of cognitive impairments consistent with the presence of dementia is lower than that suggested by neuropathological studies. The pattern of acquisition of cognitive impairments in adults with DS is similar to that seen in individuals with DAD who do not have DS.

A study of neurological changes and emotions in adults with DS yielded significant results for individuals with pathological findings on magnetic resonance imaging (MRI) and neurological examination across three scales, namely depression, indifference and pragmatic language functioning.[47] Problems of poor pragmatic language functioning appeared later in the course of suspected DAD, but not at initial testing. In these individuals, the primary emotional change was a decline in social skills such as conversational style, literal understanding and verbal expression. These emotional levels were stable over time, regardless of the degree of cognitive decline. The emotional changes were associated with abnormal findings from MRI and neurological examination. These results, together with abnormalities in brain imaging and the presence of pathological reflexes, suggested that frontal lobe dysfunction was likely to be an early manifestation of AD in DS.[47]

Another brain-imaging approach to determining the natural history of dementia in DS is to measure brain areas and memory function in prodromal phases of DAD.[48] Krasuski and colleagues found that the volumes of the right and left amygdala, hippocampus and posterior parahippocampal gyrus were positively associated with age in adults with DS without dementia.[48] Furthermore, the amygdala and hippocampal volumes correlated with memory scores.

Differential diagnosis of cognitive and functional decline

A decline in functioning in an adult with DS does not automatically mean that DAD is present. Evenhuis[49] discussed false-positive scores on the DMR in 44 adults with DS. Nearly 30% of these 44 individuals had false-positive scores. Of the false-positive results that were related to physical causes, two were due to hearing loss, and one each was due to chronic tonsillitis, depression, arthrosis, visual loss and hypothyroidism. Other conditions to consider include Parkinsonism, cerebrovascular disease, folate deficiency, vitamin B_{12} deficiency and hypercalcaemia.[50]

Hearing loss is very common. Only 7% of 90 individuals with DS had normal hearing in one study.[42] In the subgroup aged 50 years or older, only 1 out of 30 individuals (3%) had normal hearing. Van Buggenhout and colleagues examined vision and found that almost half (45%) of those aged 50 to 59 years had moderate to severe visual loss. Visual problems were common in another review of elderly patients with DS. Van Allen and colleagues[51] reported that 13 out of 20 individuals (65%) had adult-onset cataracts. Overall, 75% of elderly people with DS had visual problems. Van Allen and colleagues emphasised that even something that most middle-aged people regard as routine, namely wearing bifocals, can be problematic for many individuals with DS.

Van Buggenhout and colleagues[42] tested for thyroid dysfunction and found that nearly half of their study subjects had abnormal thyroid-stimulating hormone (TSH) levels. Most of the abnormalities were sub-clinical. The researchers found that 35% of individuals with DS aged over 50 years required treatment for hypothyroidism. Thyroid disorders in adults with DS will be discussed in detail in Chapter 7.

Burt and colleagues[52] emphasised that the extent of depressive symptoms associated with the onset of dementia in adults with DS is unclear. They studied 61 adults with DS, ranging in age from 20 to 60 years (average age 33.5 years). Their control group included 43 age-matched adults with intellectual disabilities but without DS. Burt and colleagues listed at least 15 symptoms that are common to both depression and dementia in individuals with DS. These included apathy/inactivity, loss of self-help skills, depression, urinary incontinence, irritability, slowing, being uncooperative/unmanageable, loss of housekeeping skills, greater dependency, loss of interest in surroundings, weight loss, emotional deterioration, destructive behaviour, hallucinations/delusions and sleep difficulties. They concluded that individuals with DS and depression are at increased risk of a decline in functioning. What the study could not determine was whether treatment of depression in older adults with DS reverses this functional decline.

Other differential conditions to consider are sleep apnoea and bereavement. Sleep apnoea is more common in adults with DS.[53] Folstein and Hurley[54] recommended that an evaluation of sleep apnoea should take place as part of the dementia work-up, especially if the person with DS is obese or snores loudly. Pary[55] described the case of Mr A, a 48-year-old man with DS who was referred to the clinic with probable dementia. Towards the end of the evaluation, the informants remarked that Mr A's mother had died nearly a year previously. Furthermore, Mr A had been unaware of his mother's death until several months after the funeral. Pary concluded that the functional decline disappeared following grief work, including Mr A visiting his mother's grave. Perhaps what was most remarkable about the vignette was that Mr A had severe ID and his carers were not aware that his mother's death could have much of an impact on him.

Perhaps one of the toughest differentials to untangle is that between depression and apathy associated with DAD. Landes and colleagues[45] have attempted to distinguish between the two. They list the symptoms of apathy as blunted emotional response, indifference, low social engagement, diminished initiation and poor persistence. The symptoms common to apathy and depression include diminished interest, psychomotor retardation, fatigue/hypersomnia and lack of insight. Landes and colleagues list the symptoms of depression as dysphoria, suicidal ideation, self-criticism, guilt feelings, pessimism and hopelessness. The sobering question for clinicians and researchers is 'How many adults with DS at their premorbid functioning could spontaneously voice suicidal thoughts, show self-criticism, or express guilt, pessimism or hopelessness?'

Overview of the clinical evaluation

One needs to critically examine adults with DS who present with functional decline, in order to avoid mistakenly assuming that all decline in dementia is due to DAD (as was done in the section on prevalence), and to take a cautious approach to the clinical work-up of dementia in DS. In individuals with DS, DAD is still a diagnosis of exclusion. Thus if a patient shows a functional decline and a disturbance of memory, one needs to rule out potential reversible causes before assuming that the patient has dementia. Smith[53] has previously commented that 'neuropsychologic testing and radiologic imaging do not accurately diagnose dementia or reliably [distinguish] depression from dementia.' Although Smith[53] did not provide any data for his position, his view deserves some reflection. His opinion is based on years of experience as a family practitioner with a special interest in the health problems of adults with DS. Janicki and colleagues[56] offer a variation on Smith's view. They recommend repeated evaluations to increase confidence in the diagnosis (for specific diagnostic criteria the reader should consult their article). However, the Royal College of Psychiatrists in the UK cautions that repeated psychometric or behaviour skill assessments are insufficient by themselves to diagnose dementia.[50]

The goal of the clinical evaluation of DAD in individuals with DS has not changed since clinicians first pondered the aetiology of functional decline. The aim is still to rule out all potential reversible causes. After it has been shown that reversible causes are unlikely, one can (tentatively) conclude that the person has dementia, probably of the Alzheimer type. Pary[55] reviewed the clinical evaluation and emphasised that the first step is for the family or caregiver to recognise that there may be a deterioration in functioning. Theoretically an adult with DS could request the evaluation, although the authors are unaware of this ever happening. Often the impetus for an evaluation will be a loss of bathing or eating skills, loss of social or occupational skills or a personality change. Prasher and Chung[57] advise that individuals with more severe ID may show a greater age-related decline.

The cornerstone of the initial clinical evaluation is still a history from a reliable informant and a physical examination. Ideally the informant will have had daily contact with the person for years. However, in some clinical situations the informant may be any available member of staff, regardless of their knowledge about the patient. The evaluator should insist that the informant has known the person with DS for at least one year. This recommendation is based in part on a Royal College of Psychiatrists criterion[50] that requires at least six months of symptoms and a distinct change from premorbid functioning. Table 1.1 lists the areas on which to focus during the examination.

Unfortunately, there still is no laboratory test for diagnosing DAD. Measurement of plasma levels of $A\beta1$–42 is still confined to research centres and is not yet established as a marker for AD. Brain imaging is not diagnostic, although many lay people assume that brain imaging is part of the work-up for dementia. In the absence of lateralising signs on neurological examination, one could argue that the risks of sedation outweigh the potential benefits of MRI or computerised tomography (CT). An MRI study by Prasher and colleagues[58] was terminated because of poor patient compliance (i.e. remaining still in the MRI tube) and post-procedure complications due to sedation. Blood measurements should include thyroid function tests, complete metabolic panel (electrolytes, liver enzymes, calcium, creatinine and blood urea nitrogen), a complete blood count with platelets, folate and vitamin B_{12} levels.[55]

If unlimited time and resources are available, the test battery[22] outlined above merits consideration, although one could still not definitely conclude that a patient has DAD based on a single test battery. For most clinicians, then, serial tests using the DSDS[24] or DMR[23] questionnaire are a reasonable option. Some clinicians make serial videos (over a period of years) of simple commands and find this to be quite an effective way of demonstrating dementia.

Table 1.1 Examination in adults with DS, adapted from Smith[53]

System	Possible findings
Vital signs	Arrhythmias, obesity
Ears	Impacted cerumen, hearing loss
Eyes	Visual loss, cataracts, keratoconus
Mouth	Dental abscesses, periodontal disease
Neck	Enlarged lymph nodes, enlarged thyroid gland
Lungs/back	Pneumonia, tenderness over spine or kidneys
Heart	Murmurs, arrhythmias, mitral clicks
Abdomen	Masses, enlarged liver or spleen, hypotonic bowel sounds
Musculoskeletal	Gait disturbance or muscle atrophy (spinal cord compression, atlanto-axial subluxation)
Skin	Poorly healing sores (diabetes mellitus)
Genital	Testicular cancer
Neurological	Lateralising signs, pathological reflexes, Parkinsonian signs (increased rigidity; tremor)
Mental status examination	Crying or depressed mood, responding to internal stimuli, aphasia, apraxia, agnosia, impaired memory, disorientation, alterations of consciousness, psychomotor abnormalities, compulsive behaviour

Management of individuals with Down syndrome and Alzheimer's disease

Janicki and colleagues[56] and Wilkinson and Janicki[59] have provided guidelines for managing individuals with DS and DAD. They believe that it is important to review all medications and to eliminate any unnecessary drugs. Individuals with dementia are vulnerable to delirium, and two of the commonest causes are drug interactions and excessively high drug levels. Comorbid medical conditions, such as urinary tract infections or pneumonia, should be treated. Carers must recognise safety issues such as the potential for wandering, dressing inappropriately for the weather conditions, the potential for scalding because of inability to adjust the shower or bath temperature, or swallowing difficulty and aspiration or choking on food.

There have been preliminary reports of the use of anticholinesterase inhibitors in individuals with DS and DAD (for a recent review and further information, see reports by Prasher and colleagues[60–62]).

Conclusion

As society anticipates that most people with DS will live well beyond 50 years, DAD remains a potential complication. No longer is it expected that everyone over 60 years with DS will develop clinical features of DAD. The remaining chapters of this book will review what is known about the biological correlates of AD and DS and what advances tomorrow's patients, families, caregivers and clinicians can expect.

References

1 Eyman R, Call T and White J (1991) Life expectancy in persons with Down syndrome. *Am J Ment Retard.* **95:** 603–12.

2 Yang Q, Rasmussen SA and Friedman JM (2002) Mortality associated with Down's syndrome in the USA from 1983 to 1997: a population study. *Lancet.* **359:** 1019–25.

3 Van Dyke DC, Mattheis P, Eberly SS *et al.* (eds) (1995) *Medical and Surgical Care for Children with Down Syndrome: a guide for parents.* Woodbine House, Inc., Bethesda, MD.

4 Fray MT (2000) *Caring for Kathleen: a sister's story about Down's syndrome and dementia.* British Institute of Learning Disabilities (BILD), Glasgow.

5 Holland A (2000) Ageing and learning disability. *Br J Psychiatry.* **176:** 26–31.

6 Glasson EJ, Sullivan SG, Hussain R *et al.* (2002) The changing survival profile of people with Down's syndrome: implications for genetic counselling. *Clin Genet.* **62:** 390–3.

7 Watchman K (2003) Critical issues for service planners and providers of care for people with Down's syndrome and dementia. *Br J Learn Disabil.* **31:** 81–4.

8 Zigman WB, Schupf N, Devenny DA *et al.* (2004) Incidence and prevalence of dementia in elderly adults with mental retardation without Down syndrome. *Am J Ment Retard.* **109:** 126–41.

9 Chicoine B and McGuire D (1997) Longevity of a woman with Down syndrome: a case study. *Ment Retard.* **35:** 477–9.

10 Fraser J and Mitchell A (1876) Kalmuc idiocy: report of a case with autopsy, with notes on sixty-two cases. *J Ment Sci.* **22:** 161–79.

11 Struwe F (1929) Histopathologische Untersuchungen uber Entstehung und Wesen der senilen Plaques. *Z Neurol Psychiatrie.* **122:** 291–307.

12 Lott IT (2002) Down syndrome and Alzheimer disease. In: RJ Pary (ed.) *Psychiatric Problems in Older Persons with Developmental Disabilities.* NADD Press, Kingston, NY.

13 Jervis G (1948) Early senile dementia in mongoloid idiocy. *Am J Psychiatry.* **105:** 102–6.

14 Wisniewski K, Dalton A, Crapper-McLachlan D *et al.* (1985) Alzheimer's disease in Down's syndrome: clinicopathological studies. *Neurology.* **35:** 957–61.

15 Zigman W, Schupf N, Haverman M *et al.* (1997) The epidemiology of Alzheimer disease in intellectual disability: results and recommendations from an international conference. *J Intellect Disabil Res.* **41:** 75–80.

16 Martin BA (1997) Primary care of adults with mental retardation living in the community. *Am Fam Physician.* **56:** 485–94.

17 Smith DS (1998) Down syndrome and incidence of Alzheimer's disease. *Am Fam Physician.* **57:** 1498.

18 Zigman WB, Schupf N, Sersen E *et al.* (1995) Prevalence of dementia in adults with and without Down syndrome. *Am J Ment Retard.* **100:** 403–12.

19 Prasher VP (1994) The role of cytogenetics in studies of people with Down syndrome. *J Intellect Disabil Res.* **38:** 541.

20 Bush A and Beail N (2004) Risk factors for dementia in people with Down syndrome: issues in assessment and diagnosis. *Am J Ment Retard.* **109:** 83–97.

21 Prasher VP (1999) Adaptive behavior. In: MP Janicki and AJ Dalton (eds) *Dementia, Aging, and Intellectual Disabilities: a handbook.* Brunner/Mazel, Philadelphia, PA.

22 Burt DB and Aylward EH (2000) Test battery for the diagnosis of dementia in individuals with intellectual disability. *J Intellect Disabil Res.* **44:** 175–80.

23 Evenhuis HM, Kengen MMF and Eurlings HAL (1990) *Dementia Questionnaire for Mentally Retarded Persons.* Hooge Burch Institute for Mentally Retarded People, Zwannerdam.

24 Gedye A (1995) *Dementia Scale for Down Syndrome: manual.* Gedye Research and Consulting, Vancouver, BC.

25 Reiss S (1987) *Reiss Screen for Maladaptive Behavior.* International Diagnostic Systems, Inc., Worthington, OH.

26 Bruininks RH, Woodcook RW, Weatherman RF *et al.* (1996) *Scales of Independent Behavior.* Revised Riverside, Itasca, IL.

27 Nihira K, Leland H and Lambert N (1993) *AAMR Adaptive Behavior Scales: residential and community edition.* American Association on Mental Retardation, Washington, DC.

28 Schultz J, Aman M, Kelbley T *et al.* (2004) Evaluation of screening tools for dementia in older adults with mental retardation. *Am J Ment Retard.* **109**: 98–110.

29 Lai F (1992) Alzheimer disease. In: SM Pueschel and JK Pueschel (eds) *Biomedical Concerns in Persons with Down Syndrome.* Brookes, Baltimore, MD.

30 Sekijima Y, Ikeda S, Tokuda T *et al.* (1998) Prevalence of dementia of Alzheimer type and apolipoprotein E phenotypes in aged patients with Down's syndrome. *Eur Neurol.* **39**: 234–7.

31 Visser FE, Aldenkamp AP, Van Huffelen AC *et al.* (1997) Prospective study of the prevalence of Alzheimer-type dementia in institutionalized individuals with Down syndrome. *Am J Ment Retard.* **101**: 400–12.

32 Huxley A, Prasher VP and Haque MS (2000) The dementia scale for Down's syndrome. *J Intellect Disabil Res.* **44**: 697–8.

33 Schupf N (2002) Genetic and host factors for dementia in Down's syndrome. *Br J Psychiatry.* **180**: 405–10.

34 MacDonald MLE (2004) Genetic validation of β-secretase as a drug target for Alzheimer's disease. *Clin Genet.* **65**: 458–62.

35 Schupf N, Patel B, Silverman W *et al.* (2001) Elevated plasma amyloid beta-peptide 1–42 and onset of dementia in adults with Down syndrome. *Neurosci Lett.* **301**: 199–203.

36 Mayeux R, Honig LS, Tang M-X *et al.* (2003) Plasma Aβ40 and Aβ42 and Alzheimer disease. *Neurology.* **61**: 1185–90.

37 Hattori M, Fujiyama A, Taylor TD *et al.* (2000) The DNA sequence of human chromosome 21. *Nature.* **405**: 311–19.

38 Gardiner K and Davisson M (2000) The sequence of human chromosome 21 and implications for research into Down syndrome. *Genome Biol.* 1(2) reviews 00002.1–00002.9 (epublication). www.pubmedcentral.gov/articlerender.fcgi?tool=pubmedd Pubmedid=11178230.

39 Saunders AM, Schmader K, Breitner JCS *et al.* (1993) Apolipoprotein E type 4 allele distributions in late-onset Alzheimer's disease and in other amyloid-forming diseases. *Lancet.* **342**: 710–11.

40 Thase ME, Tigner R, Smeltzer DJ and Liss L (1983) Age-related neuropsychological deficits in Down's syndrome. *Biol Psychiatry.* **19**: 571–85.

41 Evenhuis HM (1990) The natural history of dementia in Down's syndrome. *Arch Neurol.* **47**: 263–7.

42 Van Buggenhout GJCM, Trommelen JCM, Schoenmaker A *et al.* (1999) Down syndrome in a population of elderly mentally retarded patients: genetic–diagnostic survey and implications for medical care. *Am J Med Genet.* **85**: 376–84.

43 Holland AJ, Hon J, Huppert FA *et al.* (2000) Incidence and course of dementia in people with Down's syndrome: findings from a population-based study. *J Intellect Disabil Res.* **44**: 138–46.

44 Roth M, Tym E, Mountjoy CQ *et al.* (1986) CAMDEX: a standardized instrument for the diagnosis of mental disorder in the elderly, with special reference to the early detection of dementia. *Br J Psychiatry.* **149**: 698–709.

45 Landes AM, Sperry SD, Struass ME *et al.* (2001) Apathy in Alzheimer's disease. *J Am Geriatr Soc.* **49**: 1700–7.

46 Oliver C, Crayton L, Holland A *et al.* (1998) A four-year prospective study of age-related cognitive change in adults with Down's syndrome. *Psychol Med.* **28**: 1365–77.

47 Nelson LD, Orme D, Osann K *et al.* (2001) Neurological changes and emotional functioning in adults with Down syndrome. *J Intellect Disabil Res.* **45**: 450–6.

48 Krasuski JS, Alexander GE, Horwitz B *et al.* (2002) Relation of medial temporal lobe volumes to age and memory function in non-demented adults with Down's syndrome: implications for the prodromal phase of Alzheimer's disease. *Am J Psychiatry.* **159**: 74–81.

49 Evenhuis HM (1996) Further evaluation of the Dementia Questionnaire for Persons with Mental Retardation (DMR). *J Intellect Disabil Res.* **40**: 369–73.

50 Royal College of Psychiatrists (2001) *DC–LD. Diagnostic criteria for psychiatric disorders for use with adults with learning disabilities/mental retardation.* Occasional Paper No. 48. Gaskell, London.

51 Van Allen M, Fung J and Jurenka SB (1999) Health care concerns and guidelines for adults with Down syndrome. *Am J Med Genet.* **89**: 100–9.

52 Burt DB, Loveland KA and Lewis KR (1992) Depression and the onset of dementia in adults with mental retardation. *Am J Ment Retard.* **96**: 502–11.

53 Smith DS (2001) Health care management of adults with Down syndrome. *Am Fam Physician.* **64**: 1031–40.

54 Folstein MF and Hurley AD (2002) Dementia in patients with mental retardation/developmental disabilities. *Ment Health Aspects of Developmental Disabilities.* **5**: 28–31.

55 Pary RJ (2002) Down syndrome and dementia. *Ment Health Aspects of Developmental Disabilities.* **5**: 57–63.

56 Janicki MP, Hellar T, Seltzer GB *et al.* (1996) Practice guidelines for the clinical assessment and care management of Alzheimer's disease and other dementias among adults with intellectual disability. *J Intellect Disabil Res.* **40**: 374–82.

57 Prasher VP and Chung MC (1996) Causes of age-related decline in adaptive behavior of adults with Down syndrome: differential diagnoses of dementia. *Am J Ment Retard.* **101**: 175–83.

58 Prasher V, Cumelia S, Natarajan K *et al.* (2003) Magnetic resonance imaging, Down's syndrome and Alzheimer's disease: research and clinical implications. *J Intellect Disabil Res.* **47**: 90–100.

59 Wilkinson H and Janicki MP (2002) The Edinburgh Principles with accompanying guidelines and recommendations. *J Intellect Disabil Res.* **46**: 279–84.

60 Prasher VP (2004) Review of donepezil, rivastigmine, galantamine and memantine for the treatment of dementia in Alzheimer's disease in adults with Down syndrome: implications for the intellectual disability population. *Int J Geriatr Psychiatry.* **19**: 509–15.

61 Prasher VP, Fung N and Adams C (2005) Rivastigime in the treatment of dementia in Alzheimer's disease in adults with Down syndrome. *Int J Geriatr Psychiatry.* **20**: 496–7.

62 Prasher VP, Adams C and Holder R (2003) Long-term safety and efficacy of donepezil in the treatment of dementia in Alzheimer's disease in adults with Down syndrome. Open-label study. *Int J Geriatr Psychiatry.* **18**: 549–51.

Chapter 2

Neuropathology of Alzheimer's disease in Down syndrome

David M A Mann

Introduction

An association between Down syndrome (DS) and dementia was first noted by Fraser and Mitchell in 1876, who wrote that 'in not a few instances, however, death was attributed to nothing more than a general decay – a sort of precipitated senility.'[1] Since then, numerous studies[2–23] have investigated this association from both a clinical and a neuropathological standpoint, yet controversies still remain. For example, it is well recognised that many people with DS who live beyond 50 years of age display signs of mental deterioration or behavioural regression, yet relatively few of these individuals present an overt clinical deterioration that can be convincingly defined as dementia. Indeed, it is apparent that some individuals can live well into their sixth decade without showing any evidence of behavioural or cognitive decline,[23] yet as we shall see later virtually all such individuals can be expected to harbour pathology within their brains to a degree that would, in the general population, signal Alzheimer's disease (AD) both clinically and neuropathologically.

Of course, arguments about the acquisition of relevant data that reflect the burden of an additional pathological deficit upon a basic intellectual disability (ID), and the difficulties in extracting meaningful clinical data from retrospective records not specifically kept for the purpose of charting changes in cognitive function, are no doubt applicable and may go a long way towards explaining these apparent inconsistencies in many of the earlier studies. However, such arguments cannot explain the continued findings of preserved elderly people with DS in more recent prospective studies[19,20,23] of longitudinally assessed individuals. In order to explain this paradox, Wisniewski and colleagues[24,25] argued that a threshold effect might operate, dictating that a certain level of pathology must accrue within the brain in premorbidly healthy people in the general population before clinical dementia becomes apparent, and that this pathological threshold level might be higher in the DS brain. Observations that many elderly people with DS who bear the apolipoprotein (ApoE) $\epsilon2$ allele not only live longer but are also less likely to develop dementia[26–29] may point towards crucial genetic or biological differences in the capacity of individuals with DS to maintain brain function, even in the face of massive pathology. In this chapter the pathological changes that are seen in the brains of people with DS as they grow older will be reviewed, particularly with regard to how these compare with, and relate to, the changes that occur in individuals with AD within the general population.

Pathological changes in the brain in Down syndrome

Gross brain changes

The cerebral atrophy that is characteristic of AD results from the progressive effects of a pathological cascade process that ultimately leads to a shrinkage and loss of nerve cells in particular cerebral cortical and subcortical regions, and the loss of pathways connecting such areas. As a result, the weight of the brain in individuals with AD falls from a notional norm of about 1250–1450 g (varying according to age and gender) to a value that is commonly less than 1200 g, and frequently under 1000 g.

It has long been known that the brains of children and young adults with DS are not dissimilar to those of people in the general population that show distinctive gross neuropathological changes, as well as specific abnormalities of nerve cell number and neuronal connectivity. Such changes are presumably responsible for the basic ID. The brain is 'rounded' in appearance and shows a foreshortening in the anterior–posterior dimension,[30,31] with relatively small frontal lobes,[31,32] cerebellum[31] and hippocampus.[32,33] The frontal and temporal gyri, especially the superior temporal gyrus, show incomplete eversion.[30] As a result, the weight of the brain in younger individuals with DS is generally low for age compared with individuals in the general population, not usually exceeding 1250 g.[32,34–37] However, in a similar manner to that seen in AD, the brain weight in adults with DS falls after the age of 50 years, when compared with younger individuals with DS, and about 50% of individuals have a brain weight below 1000 g.[32,34–39] Morphometric analysis[40] shows that this decrease in brain size in adults with DS in later life is brought about, as in AD,[41,42] by a loss of tissue (both grey and white), especially from the posterior parts of the brain. Such changes undoubtedly relate to the onset and progression of Alzheimer-type pathology in such regions.

Serial computerised tomography (CT) scanning[43] also shows that while healthy young people with DS have smaller brains than individuals of the same age within the general population, older subjects with DS have a reduced brain size which declines further with age and upon the onset of dementia. Although their brains are smaller than usual, younger patients with DS still have normal (proportionately to size) cerebral regional glucose utilisation[44] and blood flow.[45,46] In elderly patients, as in AD, both of these parameters are reduced, particularly in the temporal and posterior parietal cortex, compared with younger individuals with DS[13] or people without DS of that age.[47]

Histological changes

Although it has long been known that many individuals with DS function less well after 40 years of age, it was not until much more recently that a link between this 'senile decay' and the presence within the brain of pathological lesions apparently identical to those seen in people in the general population suffering from AD, namely senile plaques (SP) and neurofibrillary tangles (NFT), was proposed.[48–50] Since then, the association between the presence of SP or NFT in the brains of people and DS has been rigorously investigated.[5,32,33,36–40,51–80]

Prevalence and distribution of SP and NFT

Using classic silver-staining methods, these studies[10,32,33,36–40,51–80] examined collectively the brains of 434 individuals with DS, ranging in age from under 10 years to over 70 years. Overall, the presence of SP or NFT or both was noted in 260 (60%) of these individuals. However, when analysed by decade, typical SP (see later), with or without NFT, first appeared infrequently during the second decade of life, increasing rapidly in frequency through the third and fourth decades so that nearly 100% prevalence was reported in patients aged 50–60 years and 100% in those over 60 years of age. It seems therefore that SP and NFT can be expected to develop in the brain in a predictable way if an individual with DS lives long enough. However, there have been reports of people over the age of 40 years with the DS phenotype who showed no SP or NFT.[36,62,81] It should be pointed out that in two such individuals the karyotype was not a full trisomy (a chromosomal mosaic[36] and a partial trisomy,[81] respectively) and in the others[36,62] the histological examinations were insufficiently extensive to definitely exclude the presence of SP and NFT *anywhere* in the brain. Therefore, on the basis of these limited data, it is still uncertain how often exceptions to the 'usual' association between DS and the presence of SP and NFT occur, certainly with regard to individuals with a full trisomy 21.

Furthermore, in all individuals with DS over 50 years of age, SP and NFT always seem to occur together in high numbers. However, in people under this age a much more variable picture is seen,[32,33,37,48,50,54,57,64–66,69,71,75,77,78] with many of the youngest individuals showing neither SP nor NFT, but many others aged between 30 and 40 years showing both SP and NFT in all brain areas, or in the hippocampus alone. There are yet other individuals[48,50,57,77,78] who apparently show SP alone in one or more regions. However, in no instances have NFT been reported to occur in the absence of SP.

The pattern of involvement of brain structures by SP and NFT in individuals with DS who live beyond 50 years of age[10,39,51,54,59–61,63,70,72,73,75,76,78,79] seems to closely parallel that seen in AD (for a review, the reader is referred to Mann[82]). The amygdala, hippocampus and association areas of the frontal, temporal and parietal cortex, especially the outer laminae, are all strongly affected by SP formation in DS, whereas the visual, motor and somatosensory cortex are less affected.[75,78] Nerve cells in the olfactory nuclei and tracts are likewise affected by NFT, and sometimes also by SP, in people with DS.[75,83] As in AD, typical SP are not seen in the cerebellar cortex, nor are NFT present in Purkinje cells, although occasional nerve cells of the dentate nucleus contain NFT.[80] The nucleus basalis, locus caeruleus and raphe are all severely affected by NFT in individuals with DS.[72,73,75] However, the density of SP and NFT within affected brain regions in middle-aged people with DS may differ from that in patients with AD in the general population.[38]

Comparison of SP and NFT structure in individuals with DS and AD

SP and NFT in individuals with DS generally resemble those seen in AD at both light[48,50,51,54,57] and electron[56,58,59] microscope levels. However, a high proportion of larger, more amorphous plaque cores with less compact amyloid fibrils, lacking the well-defined typical polarisation cross of AD under Congo red birefringence, has been remarked upon in older people with DS both *in vitro*[84,85] and *in situ*,[75] especially within the amygdala and entorhinal cortex.[75] However, such differences in SP morphology may only represent variations in the 'end stages' of their natural history, perhaps consequent upon a longer pathological time course in DS.

More recent immunohistochemical studies using antibodies directed against the amyloid β-peptide (Aβ) have revealed that, as in AD, in the cerebral cortex, hippocampus and amygdala in DS there are 'diffuse' types of plaques (often many more) in addition to the typical cored SP.[37,77,80,86–92] Moreover, by using end-specific antibodies that selectively recognise particular Aβ species, Aβ40 or Aβ42, it can be seen that the diffuse plaques in adults with DS (as in AD) consist mainly or even exclusively of Aβ42, whereas Aβ40 is largely present within the cored plaques.[93–96] There is also much N-terminal heterogeneity, with Aβ3(PE)–42 and Aβ11(PE)–42 being prominent species.[97–102]

Both in people with AD and in those with DS, the diffuse plaques within the cerebral cortex are not associated with a neuritic component, nor do they usually display (much) astrocytic reaction.[90,103] However, they do contain microglia,[95] the numbers of which increase in line with the amount of Aβ40.[94] Surrounding the amyloid core are various cellular and non-cellular (more Aβ) elements. Unusual accumulations of glycoproteins are present in the plaque periphery.[84,104,105] Heparan sulphate proteoglycan (HSPG) is also accumulated with the Aβ deposits within SP, both in AD and in DS,[92] as are the apolipoproteins E and J.[106] These, together with amyloid P component, complement factors and α-antichymotrypsin, act as 'chaperone' proteins,[107] promoting the β-sheet structure and mediating fibrillogenesis. Recently, a 100-kDa non-amyloidogenic protein known as AMY[108,109] or CLAC[110] has been identified by immunohistochemistry within plaques in both AD[108–110] and DS.[109,110] AMY/CLAC protein frequently, but not always, co-localises with Aβ immunostaining, and is more often present within cored, neuritic plaques than diffuse deposits. In DS, it is clearly seen that Aβ immunostaining precedes that of AMY/CLAC, with the many diffuse Aβ42 deposits being (virtually) negative for AMY/CLAC.[109,110] The significance of this non-Aβ amyloid-associated protein within the context of plaque formation and evolution remains unclear. Since AMY/CLAC protein accrues within plaques after Aβ deposition, and within Aβ40 plaques preferentially, it may play an important role in their maturation, perhaps in relation to the development of neuritic plaques or neurofibrillary changes.

Amyloid β immunostaining has also shown that, in individuals with AD, non-cortical areas such as the cerebellum[80,111–115] and striatum[111,116] contain many similarly diffuse Aβ deposits composed exclusively of Aβ42. Similar diffuse deposits are seen in these regions in adults with DS.[117] Such diffuse deposits also contain microglial cells but, in contrast to the cerebral cortical deposits, are not associated with a neuritic element, and astrocytes are only rarely present.[103]

Biochemically, the Aβ isolated from plaque cores in individuals with DS and in people with AD is identical.[84,85] Consistent with the immunohistochemical data is the finding that soluble Aβ extractable from DS brains is composed mainly of Aβ species terminating at amino acid 42,[118] although there is considerable N-terminal heterogeneity, with full-length Aβ1–42 and truncated species Aβ3(PE)–42 being most prominent. Indeed, the proportion of the latter peptide species increases with age, and it becomes the predominant peptide species within plaques as the pathological process progresses.[101,102,119] These time-associated modifications of the N-terminus of Aβ peptide may render the amyloid deposits less susceptible to degradation by aminopeptidase and facilitate their transformation into cored deposits.

Amyloid β is also present within the walls of arteries that exhibit a so-called 'congophilic angiopathy.'[120–122] A heavy deposition of Aβ protein within the walls of large meningeal arteries, especially those supplying the posterior hemispheres and cerebellum, and within the walls of some intraparenchymal arteries, is also a feature of most middle-aged individuals with DS.[80] Glenner and Wong[121] have shown that Aβ of blood vessels in DS is biochemically identical to that in arterial walls in AD, and immunohistochemistry shows this to be largely composed of Aβ40. This vascular amyloidosis is also associated with the deposition of HSPG both in adults from the general population with AD and in adults with DS.[91]

Immunohistochemistry[123–127] and direct protein sequencing[127–129] indicate that the microtubule-associated protein, tau, is the major antigenic determinant of the paired helical filaments (PHF) of the NFT in AD, although ubiquitin protein also forms an important part of the structure.[130–133] Lectin histochemistry[104,105,134] shows that NFT in AD contain, or are at least associated with, certain saccharide sequences. These immunohistochemical findings with regard to tau and ubiquitin also apply in DS,[90,135] although in individuals with DS the NFT do not appear to interact with lectins (Mann *et al.*, unpublished data). Immunoblotting[136,137] shows similar mobility profiles for tau proteins in the brains of elderly individuals with DS to those in AD. Immunohistochemical evidence for caspase activation in NFT-bearing neurons and dystrophic neurites both in AD[138,139] and in individuals with DS[139,140] suggests a role for apoptotic pathways in the neurodegenerative process.

Other pathological changes

As in AD, a granulovacuolar degeneration of neurons in the hippocampus, particularly in area CA1, is a feature of DS in middle age,[51,54,57,59,65] and Hirano bodies are also common in this part of the hippocampus.[57,59] As with NFT, the granular component in granulovacuolar degeneration exhibits caspase-3 activity,[141] which again suggests that an apoptotic mechanism is operating in cells affected by this pathology.

Patients with AD often show mild extrapyramidal signs late in the course of the illness, associated with mild loss of cells from the substantia nigra. This is usually due to neurofibrillary degeneration, and nigral cells containing Lewy bodies are mostly absent. Similar changes are also found in elderly DS subjects.[142–145] However, investigations using antibodies to α-synuclein (the major protein component of Lewy bodies) have shown that Lewy bodies are commonplace within the amygdala and entorhinal cortex of patients with familial AD due to amyloid precursor protein (APP) and presenilin mutations, but are rare in sporadic AD.[146,147] Similarly, Lewy bodies are commonly present within these same brain regions (but not in the cerebral cortex) in many elderly people with DS.[148]

Calcification of the walls of the larger arteries and deposition of calcified deposits (calcospherites) around capillaries of the globus pallidus are often seen in late-onset cases of AD,[149] and elderly individuals with DS also show excessive calcification of this part of the basal ganglia.[149–151] However, it is unclear whether this change is related to ageing alone or whether the additional burden of AD pathology has a bearing on its frequent occurrence.

Neuronal fallout and neurochemical changes in Down syndrome

Because of developmental deficiencies, it is unlikely that individuals with DS start life with the same complement of nerve cells as their non-DS counterparts in the general population. There seems to be a low (for age) number of nerve cells in temporal[38,71,76] and other areas of the cortex,[6,71,152,153] hippocampus,[65] subcortex and brainstem.[38,71,154–156] Abnormalities in dendritic spines,[79,157–160] arrested synaptogenesis[10,153] and delayed postnatal myelination[161] have all been reported. All of these structural changes are likely to result from abnormal modelling and wiring of the brain caused by a failure to properly integrate and coordinate the many growth and transcription factors that come into play at different stages during the developmental and maturational periods of brain growth. Indeed, several transcription factors are encoded on chromosome 21, such as Ets-2 (see later). However, despite gene triplication, Ets-2 levels do not appear to be overexpressed in the brains of individuals with DS.[162,163] Ets-2 requires cooperation with other transcription factors such as Fos and Jun for activation; JunD levels are low in DS brain,[164] whereas Fos levels are increased.[165] Disordering of the complex relationships involving these and perhaps other transcription factors may therefore underpin some of the developmental abnormalities, and may contribute to the later development of Alzheimer-type pathology.

Thus it cannot be assumed prima facie that 'low values' for cell number represent actual loss of cell complement in elderly people with DS associated with the development of Alzheimer-type pathology. However, when cell counts in elderly individuals with DS are compared with those from young individuals with DS,[39,76] it is apparent that an actual loss and atrophy of nerve cells in many brain regions does indeed occur. In elderly people with DS there is loss of pyramidal[72] and non-pyramidal[166] nerve cells from areas of the temporal cortex, hippocampus[65] and entorhinal cortex.[167] The corpus callosum is thinned, consistent with loss of neocortical and hippocampal neurons.[168] The nucleus basalis,[70,73,155,169] locus caeruleus,[70,73,170,171] dorsal raphe[70,73] and ventral tegmentum[142,146] are also grossly depleted of nerve cells. Atrophy of surviving nerve cells of these types also takes place, as evidenced by a reduction in nucleolar size (an index of ribosomal RNA synthesis and cellular protein synthetic activity).[70,72,73,76] This pattern of cell loss and atrophy is similar to that in AD, as compared with people of similar age in the general population (for a review, the reader is referred to Mann[82]).

In AD, nerve cell atrophy and loss lead to associated reductions in neurochemical markers (i.e. transmitter levels, enzyme activities or receptor densities).[172] In elderly individuals with DS, as would be anticipated, low levels of choline acetyltransferase (ChAT) within the cerebral cortex and other brain regions have been reported.[69,173,174] Noradrenaline[69,174–176] and 5-hydroxytryptamine[174,177] levels are reduced in the cortex and other areas. Loss of glutamate and γ-aminobutyric acid[178] from cerebral cortex has been reported, as has a reduction in D-^{3}H-aspartate binding.[179] Dopamine levels appear to be unaltered.[69,174] Somatostatin levels also appear to be low in the brains of elderly people with DS.[180]

Thus, in general, differences in SP and NFT structure or chemistry between the brains of individuals with AD and and those with DS seem to be minor, and the patterns of neuronal damage and loss of transmitters also appear to be similar. Any variations that may possibly occur might reflect differences in patients' life history (e.g. community *vs.* institutionalised life) or the different time courses of evolution of pathology, and may not necessarily be of major aetiological or pathogenetic significance. Moreover, the changes of AD in elderly patients with DS are not due to mental handicap per se. Malamud[55] found that although AD changes were present in all patients with DS over 40 years of age, these occurred in other (non-DS) intellectually disabled people at a prevalence rate similar to that seen in individuals of the same age in the general population.

The time course of pathological events

The predictability with which the pathological changes of AD develop in elderly people with DS has made it possible to reconstruct a chronological course of pathological events by pooling cross-sectional data from young and old individuals with DS, and to follow them in time to that end-point which is characteristically seen at autopsy in individuals in the general population dying from AD itself. Such studies provide a unique opportunity to determine the earliest tissue changes of the destructive process of AD in humans. This kind of study cannot be performed on patients with AD itself, as in these cases brain tissues are only usually available at post-mortem, mostly from clinical and pathological 'end-stage' cases in whom the early changes of the disease either will no longer be present, or will not be easily identifiable. Moreover, it is not easy to replicate these studies in the non-demented elderly population, as it is difficult to distinguish those (non-demented) individuals who show early pathological stages of AD and who would have gone on to develop clinical AD from other patients who also show such minimal changes, but who might not necessarily have developed the full-blown pathological picture of AD, and become demented, had they lived longer.

Therefore such chronological studies in DS,[37,77,80,86–90,92,96,103,106,135,181–185] using immunohistochemical probes to detect the presence of molecular and cellular elements such as Aβ, tau, ubiquitin, PHF, oligosaccharides, proteoglycans, apolipoproteins, complement factors or glial cells, have shown that the sequence of changes within the cerebral cortex and hippocampus is initiated by deposition of Aβ protein. This is deposited as Aβ42(43), in the form of diffuse plaques, but there is some N-terminal heterogeneity, even in these early deposits, with Aβ3(PE)–42 and Aβ11(PE)–42 being prominent species.[97–102] The latter species become increasingly common as the plaques evolve over time, and racemisation and isomerisation may occur, particularly involving aspartate residues at positions 1 and 7.[98,99,186–188] Amyloid β deposition can commence in DS during the early teens or sometimes even earlier. Usually the cerebral cortex (particularly the parahippocampal, inferior and middle temporal gyri) is affected before the hippocampal formation.

Soon afterwards activated microglial cells are present within Aβ deposits, and accumulations of glycoconjugates, apolipoproteins, complement factors, HSPG and other granular material detectable by anti-ubiquitin appear as the Aβ becomes fibrillar and the plaque begins to 'mature.' Later, cored amyloid deposits containing more activated microglia, much complement, apolipoproteins, ubiquitinated material and larger quantities of oligosaccharide and HSPG are seen. These cored deposits are reactive with anti-tau and anti-acid glial filament protein and contain filamentous structures (PHF) that are immunoreactive with anti-ubiquitin. At this stage, NFT are only occasionally present in the cerebral cortex, but are usually numerous in the hippocampus, especially in area CA1 and the subiculum, entorhinal cortex and amygdala. After 50 years of age a pathological picture indistinguishable from that of AD is seen. Deposition of Aβ within the cerebellar cortex occurs about 5 years later than that in the cerebral cortex, although such deposits never become associated with a neuritic change, nor do NFT appear in Purkinje or other cerebellar cortical cells.

Therefore it seems that the onset and progression of the pathological cascade of AD in individuals with DS are triggered by events that lead to deposition of Aβ protein within the cerebral cortex. However, characteristic of the pathological process in DS is the prolonged prodromal period of as much as 25 years during which there is progressive formation of diffuse Aβ deposits with minimal or no fibrillisation of the Aβ protein, no neuronal loss and few or no neurofibrillary changes. What impact, if any, these early diffuse plaques might have on brain function is unclear, and it has yet to be determined whether they have any clinical repercussions. Functional impairment in later life seems to relate to the appearance and progress of neuritic plaques and neurofibrillary tangles, changes that undoubtedly lead to neuronal dysfunction and death, together with a loss of connectivity within the brain.

Causative factors

Although the pathological changes that are seen in the brains of individuals with DS and in people with AD may appear to be essentially identical, the fundamental mechanisms that drive the destructive process in each condition are likely to be different. It is widely believed that in AD the pathological cascade is triggered by the deposition of Aβ, although there are various 'routes' into this, some relating to autosomal-dominant mutations in APP[189–192] and presenilin genes[193] that favour a mismetabolism of APP and lead to overproduction[194] and excessive deposition[195–198] of Aβ, especially Aβ42(43). About 95% of individuals with DS have a full trisomy 21 and as such will have three, rather than two, full copies of chromosome 21, including the APP gene itself located on that chromosome. In DS, because of the triplication of chromosome 21 the APP gene is overexpressed by around four- to fivefold.[89,199–201] Therefore imbalances in the handling of such overproduction of APP may, in an analogous way to AD, 'feed' the β/γ-secretase cleavage pathway, leading to early and progressive deposition of Aβ. The finding of an increase in the ratio of Aβ42 to Aβ40 in DS brain, even from a very early age before plaques appear within the brain, would be consistent with this.[118]

However, around 4–6% of individuals with phenotypical DS are 'translocational', with only a partial triplication of chromosome 21, usually the most distal part of the long arm obligatory for expression of the DS phenotype. In the remaining 1% of individuals, a mosaic chromosomal abnormality is present in which only a proportion of the body's cells carry the trisomy. Whether and to what extent these translocational or mosaical patients also show Alzheimer-type changes is unclear. In one study[81] a woman with a partial trisomy karyotype,

46,XX,rec(21)dup q, inv(21) (p12q22.1), exhibited all the physical features of DS and although her brain showed the typical developmental defects of DS, no significant tau or Aβ deposition was seen. Fluorescence *in-situ* hybridisation analysis showed that the APP gene was present as two copies, whereas genes within the DS 'critical region' were present in triplicate. This important case provides further support for the view that the development of AD in DS is due to the presence of the additional copy of the APP gene. There have also been two reports of the presence of Alzheimer-type pathology in the brains of mosaic DS individuals,[202,203] which suggests that even incomplete trisomy can be sufficient to induce the pathological cascade.

To date, therefore, it seems that the pathological cascade of AD is triggered by deposition in the brain of Aβ which, in DS and at least in some inherited forms of AD, is a consequence of excessive production and catabolism of APP. Whether it is Aβ itself that is neurotoxic and responsible for subsequent pathological events is still far from clear. Certainly there is a wealth of experimental data pointing towards roles for Aβ in the generation of free radicals and oxidative stress, apoptosis and excitotoxicity. None of these are proven within the human brain, and it is still possible that deposition of Aβ may simply represent a relatively innocuous tissue marker of a wider-ranging process that carries in its wake other changes which cause the 'malignant' neurofibrillary alterations and eventual cell death. Indeed, it is clear that deposition of Aβ per se does not always lead to neuritic changes and NFT formation in both AD and DS, particularly in areas such as the striatum[116] and cerebellum.[80,112] If it is responsible, Aβ may have to adopt a particular physico-chemical form in order to exert toxicity, or there may be differential vulnerabilities among neuronal populations that put certain cortical or subcortical neurons at greatest risk.

However, it must be remembered that triplication of chromosome 21 may involve the overexpression of many other genes, and these could also potentially have an impact on the causation or progression of the pathological changes. Among them is the Cu/Zn-superoxide dismutase-1 (SOD1) gene. A number of studies have shown SOD1 to be elevated in a variety of cell types and organs, including brain, in both young and elderly individuals with DS, consistent with the extra gene copy.[204–207] This could play a part in the generation of oxidative cell damage (see below). Again the translocational DS case described by Prasher,[81] in which there was no Alzheimer-type pathology and the SOD1 gene was not duplicated, illustrates the potential involvement of this gene in the pathogenetic cascade.

Similarly, the gene for the neurotrophic factor S-100β, which is produced by astrocytes, maps to chromosome 21, and both S-100β and its message are increased in young DS brain,[208,209] as are the numbers of S-100β immunoreactive astrocytes.[210] S-100β can induce expression of APP,[211] and may therefore exacerbate the increase in APP expression due to the possession of the extra gene copy per se. Thus excessive production of S-100β by astrocytes and excessive astrocytic activity may potentiate the formation and deposition of Aβ, and promote neuritic changes.[212] However, in the above-mentioned translocational DS case,[81] the S-100β gene was triplicated, yet no significant AD pathology (including astrocytic changes) was present, even though this individual lived to 78 years of age. Such findings would argue that the S-100β pathology seen in trisomy 21 DS is likely to be reactive to the presence of Aβ deposition, rather than causing it.

Furthermore, the Aβ-producing enzyme β-secretase, 'beta-site amyloid precursor protein-cleaving enzyme' (BACE-2), is also encoded on chromosome 21. Elevated levels of BACE-2 have been detected in the brain in individuals with DS,[213] and BACE-2 immunoreactivity has been detected in NFT-bearing but not in non-NFT-bearing neurons in DS.[214] Therefore overactivity (and overexpression) of BACE-2 may contribute, in conjunction with overexpression of the APP gene, to the extensive and earlier deposition of Aβ in DS.

Lastly, the gene for the transcription factor Ets-2, which is located on chromosome 21q22.3 and therefore triplicated in DS, may be a contributory factor. Ets-2 acts as a transcriptional regulator for APP[215] and may therefore act in concert to further elevate APP expression (by 1.5 times) beyond that which might be expected for triplication of the APP gene alone – a three- to fourfold increase in APP expression has been detected in DS.[89] However, it is unclear whether Ets-2 is indeed overexpressed in DS, as conflicting results have been obtained.[162,163]

However, most AD is not inherited in a 'simple' Mendelian fashion but represents a complex interaction between various genes and probably environmental factors as well. The strongest genetic factor associated to date with late-onset sporadic and familial AD is the ApoE gene. This is a polymorphic gene that occurs in three major allelic forms known as ε2, ε3 and ε4. In AD there is overrepresentation of the ε4 allele,[216] which is increased from a normal population level of around 14% to 30–50% depending on the study and ethnic group. Most studies have shown that the ApoE ε4 allele frequency in DS does not differ from that in controls.[26–29,94,217–227] Indeed, the ε4 allele frequency in elderly individuals with DS has been reported to be significantly lower than that in age-matched controls, which suggests premature death of bearers of this allele.[27,226,227] Conversely, as in AD,[228] bearers of the ApoE ε2 allele with DS live longer, and are less likely to become demented.[26–29] In AD there is a gene–dosage effect on deposition of Aβ40 with increasing number of ApoE ε4 alleles,[229,230] although in DS neither Aβ40 nor Aβ42(43) levels varied, regardless of whether the ε4 allele was present or not[95] (*see* Chapter 3 for further details).

Late-onset AD has been (variably) associated with increased frequencies of common polymorphisms in either the presenilin 1 (PS1) gene[231] or the α-1-antichymotrypsin (ACT) gene.[232] Polymorphisms in these two genes have been examined in DS,[233] but neither of them showed an increased frequency compared with controls, nor did the frequencies differ in demented compared with non-demented individuals with DS.

Conclusion

Present evidence suggests that individuals with DS suffer exactly the same pathological process in later life as individuals with AD in the general population. There is nothing of substance to distinguish the pathological changes in either condition. However, it is likely that the triggers for the pathological cascade differ in the two conditions. In DS, triplication of chromosome 21, and of the APP gene in particular, seems to be critical, and leads to overproduction of APP, which in turn 'feeds' the amyloidogenic pathways of the brain and promotes the amyloid cascade process. In AD the same pathological route is followed, although here the factors that cause or promote this cascade are diverse, with those forms of the disease that are associated with autosomal-dominant mutations in APP or presenilin genes mirroring the pathogenetic process of DS most closely. Studies of the pathology of DS at different stages of life have already proved instrumental in unravelling many of the mysteries of the process of AD, and because of the near certainty of development of pathology, studies in DS will continue to serve, even in this era of cell and animal transgenesis, as the best and most 'natural' of models of AD within the wider population.

References

1 Fraser J and Mitchell A (1876) Kalmuc idiocy: report of a case with autopsy, with notes on sixty-two cases. *J Ment Sci.* **22**: 161–9.
2 Owens D, Dawson JC and Losin S (1971) Alzheimer's disease in Down's syndrome. *Am J Ment Defic.* **75**: 606–12.
3 Dalton AJ, Crapper DR and Schlotterer CR (1974) Alzheimer's disease in Down's syndrome: visual retention deficits. *Cortex.* **10**: 366–77.
4 Wisniewski KE, Howe J, Gwyn-Williams D *et al.* (1978) Precocious ageing and dementia in patients with Down's syndrome. *Biol Psychiatry.* **13**: 619–27.
5 Lott IT and Lai F (1982) Dementia in Down's syndrome: observations from a neurology clinic. *Appl Res Ment Retard.* **3**: 233–9.
6 Miniszek NA (1983) Development of Alzheimer's disease in Down's syndrome individuals. *Am J Ment Defic.* **87**: 377–85.
7 Dalton AJ and Crapper DR (1984) Incidence of memory deterioration in ageing persons with Down's syndrome. In: JM Berg (ed.) *Perspectives and Progress in Mental Retardation. Volume 2.* University Park Press, Baltimore, MD.
8 Thase ME, Tigner R, Smeltzer D *et al.* (1984) Age-related neuropsychological deficits in Down's syndrome. *Biol Psychiatry.* **19**: 571–85.
9 Hewitt KE, Carter G and Jancar J (1985) Ageing in Down's syndrome. *Br J Psychiatry.* **147**: 58–62.
10 Wisniewski KE, Dalton AJ, Crapper-McLachlan DR *et al.* (1985) Alzheimer's disease in Down's syndrome. Clinicopathologic studies. *Neurology.* **35**: 957–61.
11 Dalton AJ and Crapper-McLachlan DR (1986) Clinical expression of Alzheimer's disease in Down's syndrome. *Psychiatr Clin North Am.* **4**: 659–70.
12 Schapiro MB, Haxby JV, Grady CL *et al.* (1986) Cerebral glucose utilization, quantitative tomography and cognitive function in adult Down's syndrome. In: CJ Epstein (ed.) *Neurobiology of Down's Syndrome.* Raven Press, New York.
13 Wisniewski KE, Laure-Kamionowska M, Connell F *et al.* (1986) Neuronal density and synaptogenesis in the postnatal stage of brain maturation in Down's syndrome. In: CJ Epstein (ed.) *The Neurobiology of Down's Syndrome.* Raven Press, New York.
14 Fenner ME, Hewitt KE and Torpy DM (1987) Down's syndrome: intellectual and behavioural functioning during adulthood. *J Ment Defic Res.* **31**: 241–9.
15 Zigman WB, Schupf N, Lubin RA *et al.* (1987) Premature regression of adults with Down's syndrome. *Am J Ment Defic.* **92**: 161–8.
16 Silverstein AB, Herbs D and Miller TJ (1988) Effects of age on the adaptive behaviour of institutionalized and non-institutionalized individuals with Down's syndrome. *Am J Ment Retard.* **92**: 455–60.
17 Lai F and Williams RA (1989) Alzheimer's disease in Down's syndrome. *Neurology.* **37**: 332–9.
18 Evenhuis HM (1990) The natural history of dementia in Down's syndrome. *Arch Neurol.* **47**: 263–7.
19 Burt DB, Loveland KA, Chen Y-W *et al.* (1995) Aging in adults with Down syndrome: report from a longitudinal study. *Am J Ment Retard.* **100**: 262–70.

20 Devenny DA, Silverman WP, Hill AL *et al.* (1996) Normal ageing in adults with Down's syndrome: a longitudinal study. *J Intellect Disabil Res.* **40**: 208–21.

21 Zigman WB, Schupf N, Sersen E *et al.* (1996) Prevalence of dementia in adults with and without Down's syndrome. *Am J Ment Retard.* **100**: 403–12.

22 Holland AJ, Hon J, Huppert FA *et al.* (1998) Population-based study of the prevalence and presentation of dementia in adults with Down's syndrome. *Br J Psychiatry.* **172**: 493–8.

23 Devenny DA, Krinsky-McHale SJ, Sersen G *et al.* (2000) Sequence of cognitive decline in dementia in adults with Down's syndrome. *J Intellect Disabil Res.* **44**: 654–65.

24 Wisniewski HM and Rabe A (1986) Discrepancy between Alzheimer-type neuropathology and dementia in persons with Down's syndrome. *Ann NY Acad Sci.* **477**: 247–60.

25 Wisniewski HM, Rabe A and Wisniewski KE (1987) Neuropathology and dementia in people with Down's syndrome. In: *Banbury Report No. 27. Molecular Neuropathology of Ageing.* Cold Spring Harbor Laboratory Press, Plainview, NY.

26 Royston MC, Mann D, Pickering-Brown S *et al.* (1994) Apolipoprotein E ε2 allele promotes longevity and protects patients with Down's syndrome from dementia. *Neuroreport.* **5**: 2583–5.

27 Tyrrell J, Cosgrave M, Hawi Z *et al.* (1998) A protective effect of apolipoprotein E ε2 allele on dementia in Down's syndrome. *Biol Psychiatry.* **43**: 397–400.

28 Lambert J-C, Perez-Tur J, Dupire M-J *et al.* (1996) Analysis of Apo E alleles impact in Down's syndrome. *Neurosci Lett.* **220**: 57–60.

29 Rubinsztein DC, Hon J, Stevens F *et al.* (1999) Apo E genotypes and risk of dementia in Down syndrome. *Am J Med Genet.* **88**: 344–7.

30 Davidoff LM (1928) The brain in mongolian idiocy. *Arch Neurol Psychiatry.* **20**: 1229–57.

31 Crome L and Stern J (1972) *Pathology of Mental Retardation* (2e). Williams & Wilkins, Baltimore, MD.

32 Wisniewski KE, Wisniewski HM and Wen GY (1985) Occurrence of neuropathological changes and dementia of Alzheimer's disease in Down's syndrome. *Ann Neurol.* **17**: 278–82.

33 Sylvester PE (1983) The hippocampus in Down's syndrome. *J Ment Defic Res.* **27**: 227–36.

34 Benda CE (1960) *The Child with Mongolism (Congenital Acromicria).* Grune & Stratton, New York.

35 Solitaire GB and Lamarche JB (1967) Brain weight in the adult mongol. *J Ment Defic Res.* **11**: 79–84.

36 Whalley LJ (1982) The dementia of Down's syndrome and its relevance to aetiological studies of Alzheimer's disease. *Ann N Y Acad Sci.* **396**: 39–53.

37 Mann DMA and Esiri MM (1989) Regional acquisition of plaques and tangles in Down's syndrome patients under 50 years of age. *J Neurol Sci.* **89**: 169–79.

38 Mann DMA (1988) Neuropathological association between Down's syndrome and Alzheimer's disease. *Mech Ageing Dev.* **43**: 99–136.

39 Mann DMA, Royston MC and Ravindra CR (1990) Some morphometric observations on the brains of patients with Down's syndrome: their relationship to age and dementia. *J Neurol Sci.* **99**: 153–64.

40 De La Monte SM and Hedley-White ET (1990) Small cerebral hemispheres in adults with Down's syndrome. Contributions of developmental arrest and lesions of Alzheimer's disease. *J Neuropathol Exp Neurol.* **49**: 509–20.

41 De La Monte S (1989) Quantitation of cerebral atrophy in preclinical and end-stage Alzheimer's disease. *Ann Neurol.* **25**: 450–9.

42 Mann DMA (1991) The topographic distribution of brain atrophy in Alzheimer's disease. *Acta Neuropathol.* **83**: 81–6.

43 Schapiro MB, Luxemberg JS, Kaye JA *et al.* (1989) Serial quantitative CT analysis of brain morphometrics in adult Down's syndrome at different ages. *Neurology.* **39:** 1349–53.

44 Schapiro MB, Grady CL, Kumar A *et al.* (1990) Regional cerebral glucose metabolism is normal in young adults with Down's syndrome. *J Cereb Blood Flow Metab.* **10:** 199–206.

45 Risberg J (1980) Regional cerebral blood flow measurements by ^{133}Xe inhalation: methodology and application in neuropathology and psychiatry. *Brain Lang.* **9:** 9–34.

46 Schapiro MB, Berman KF, Friedland RP *et al.* (1988) Regional blood flow is not reduced in young adult with Down's syndrome. *Ann Neurol.* **24:** 310.

47 Melamed E, Mildworf B, Sharav T *et al.* (1987) Regional cerebral blood flow in Down's syndrome. *Ann Neurol.* **22:** 275–8.

48 Struwe F (1929) Histopathologische Untersuchungen uber Enstehung und Wesen der senilen plaques. *Z Neurol Psychiatrie.* **122:** 291–307.

49 Bertrand I and Koffas D (1946) Case d'idiotie mongolienne adult avec nombreuses plaques seniles et concretions calcaires pallidales. *Rev Neurol (Paris).* **78:** 338–45.

50 Jervis GA (1948) Early senile dementia and mongoloid idiocy. *Am J Psychiatry.* **105:** 102–6.

51 Solitaire GB and Lamarche JB (1966) Alzheimer's disease and senile dementia as seen in mongoloids: neuropathological observations. *Am J Ment Defic.* **70:** 840–8.

52 Neumann NA (1967) Langdon Down syndrome and Alzheimer's disease. *J Neuropathol Exp Neurol.* **26:** 149–50.

53 Haberland C (1969) Alzheimer's disease in Down's syndrome: clinical and neuropathological observations. *Acta Neurol Belg.* **69:** 369–80.

54 Olson MI and Shaw CM (1969) Presenile dementia and Alzheimer's disease in mongolism. *Brain.* **92:** 147–56.

55 Malamud N (1972) Neuropathology of organic brain syndromes associated with ageing. In: CM Gaitz (ed.) *Ageing and the Brain. Advances in Behavioural Biology. Volume 3.* Plenum Press, New York.

56 O'Hara PT (1972) Electron microscopical study of the brain in Down's syndrome. *Brain.* **95:** 681–4.

57 Burger PC and Vogel FS (1973) The development of the pathological changes of Alzheimer's disease and senile dementia in patients with Down's syndrome. *Am J Pathol.* **73:** 457–76.

58 Schochet SS, Lampert PW and McCormick WF (1973) Neurofibrillary tangles in patients with Down's syndrome: a light and electron microscope study. *Acta Neuropathol.* **23:** 342–6.

59 Ellis WG, McCulloch JR and Corley CL (1974) Presenile dementia in Down's syndrome. Ultrastructural identity with Alzheimer's disease. *Neurology.* **24:** 101–6.

60 Reid AH and Maloney AFJ (1974) Giant cell arteritis and arteriolitis associated with amyloid angiopathy in an elderly mongol. *Acta Neuropathol.* **27:** 131–7.

61 Crapper DR, Dalton AJ, Skoptiz M *et al.* (1975) Alzheimer degeneration in Down's syndrome. *Arch Neurol.* **32:** 618–23.

62 Murdoch JC and Adams H (1977) Reply to W Hughes (1977) Atherosclerosis, Down's syndrome and Alzheimer's disease. *BMJ.* **2:** 702.

63 Rees S (1977) The incidence of ultrastructural abnormalities in the cortex of two retarded human brains (Down's syndrome). *Acta Neuropathol.* **37:** 65–8.

64 Wisniewski KE, Jervis GA, Moretz RC *et al.* (1979) Alzheimer neurofibrillary tangles in diseases other than senile and presenile dementia. *Ann Neurol.* **5:** 288–94.

65 Ball MJ and Nuttall K (1980) Neurofibrillary tangles and granulovacuolar degeneration and neurone loss in Down's syndrome: quantitative comparison with Alzheimer's dementia. *Ann Neurol.* **7:** 462–5.

66 Ropper AH and Williams RS (1980) Relationship between plaques and tangles and dementia in Down's syndrome. *Neurology.* **30**: 739–44.

67 Blumbergs P, Beran R and Hicks P (1981) Myoclonus in Down's syndrome: association with Alzheimer's disease. *Arch Neurol.* **38**: 453–4.

68 Pogacar S and Rubio A (1982) Morphological features of Pick's and atypical Alzheimer's disease in Down's syndrome. *Acta Neuropathol.* **58**: 249–54.

69 Yates CM, Simpson A, Gordon A *et al.* (1983) Catecholamines and cholinergic enzymes in presenile and senile Alzheimer-type dementia and Down's syndrome. *Brain Res.* **280**: 119–26.

70 Mann DMA, Yates PO and Marcyniuk B (1984) Alzheimer's presenile dementia, senile dementia of Alzheimer type and Down's syndrome in middle age from an age-related continuum of pathological changes. *Neuropathol Appl Neurobiol.* **10**: 185–207.

71 Ross MH, Galaburda AM and Kemper TL (1984) Down's syndrome: is there a decreased population of neurones? *Neurology.* **34**: 909–16.

72 Mann DMA, Yates PO and Marcyniuk B (1985) Some morphometric observations on the cerebral cortex and hippocampus in presenile Alzheimer's disease, senile dementia of Alzheimer type and Down's syndrome in middle age. *J Neurol Sci.* **69**: 139–59.

73 Mann DMA, Yates PO, Marcyniuk B *et al.* (1985) Pathological evidence for neurotransmitter deficits in Down's syndrome of middle age. *J Ment Defic Res.* **29**: 125–35.

74 Belza MG and Urich H (1986) Cerebral amyloid angiopathy in Down's syndrome. *Clin Neuropathol.* **6**: 257–60.

75 Mann DMA, Yates PO, Marcyniuk B *et al.* (1986) The topography of plaques and tangles in Down's syndrome patients of different ages. *Neuropathol Appl Neurobiol.* **12**: 447–57.

76 Mann DMA, Yates PO, Marcyniuk B *et al.* (1987) Loss of nerve cells from cortical and subcortical areas in Down's syndrome patients at middle age: quantitative comparisons with younger Down's patients and patients with Alzheimer's disease. *J Neurol Sci.* **80**: 79–89.

77 Giaccone G, Tagliavini F, Linoli G *et al.* (1989) Down patients: extracellular pre-amyloid deposits precede neuritic degeneration and senile plaques. *Neurosci Lett.* **9**: 232–8.

78 Motte J and Williams RS (1989) Age-related changes in the density and morphology of plaques and neurofibrillary tangles in Down's syndrome brains. *Acta Neuropathol.* **77**: 535–46.

79 Ferrer I and Gullotta F (1990) Down's syndrome and Alzheimer's disease: dendritic spine counts in the hippocampus. *Acta Neuropathol.* **79**: 680–5.

80 Mann DMA, Jones D, Prinja D *et al.* (1990) The prevalence of amyloid (A4) protein deposits within the cerebral and cerebellar cortex in Alzheimer's disease and Down's syndrome. *Acta Neuropathol.* **80**: 318–27.

81 Prasher VP, Farrer MJ, Kessling AM *et al.* (1998) Molecular mapping of Alzheimer-type dementia in Down's syndrome. *Ann Neurol.* **43**: 380–3.

82 Mann DMA (1985) The neuropathology of Alzheimer's disease: a review with pathogenetic, aetiological and therapeutic considerations. *Mech Ageing Dev.* **31**: 213–55.

83 Mann DMA, Tucker CM and Yates PO (1988) Alzheimer's disease: an olfactory connection? *Mech Ageing Dev.* **42**: 1–15.

84 Masters CL, Simms G, Weinmann NA *et al.* (1985) Amyloid plaque core protein in Alzheimer's disease and Down's syndrome. *Proc Natl Acad Sci USA.* **82**: 4245–9.

85 Allsop D, Kidd M, Landon M *et al.* (1986) Isolated senile plaque cores in Alzheimer's disease and Down's syndrome show differences in morphology. *J Neurol Neurosurg Psychiatry.* **49**: 886–92.

86 Allsop D, Haga S-I, Haga C *et al.* (1989) Early senile plaques in Down's syndrome brains show a close relationship with cell bodies of neurones. *Neuropathol Appl Neurobiol.* **15**: 531–42.

87 Ikeda S-I, Yanagisawa N, Allsop D *et al.* (1989) Evidence of amyloid β protein immunoreactive early plaque lesions in Down's syndrome brains. *Lab Invest.* **61:** 133–7.

88 Mann DMA, Brown AMT, Prinja D *et al.* (1989) An analysis of the morphology of senile plaques in Down's syndrome patients of different ages using immunocytochemical and lectin histochemical methods. *Neuropathol Appl Neurobiol.* **15:** 317–29.

89 Rumble B, Retallack R, Hilbich C *et al.* (1989) Amyloid (A4) protein and its precursor in Down's syndrome and Alzheimer's disease. *NEJM.* **320:** 1446–52.

90 Murphy GM, Eng LF, Ellis WG *et al.* (1990) Antigenic profile of plaques and neurofibrillary tangles in the amygdala in Down's syndrome: a comparison with Alzheimer's disease. *Brain Res.* **537:** 102–8.

91 Spargo E, Luthert PJ, Anderton BH *et al.* (1990) Antibodies raised against different portions of A4 protein identify a subset of plaques in Down's syndrome. *Neurosci Lett.* **115:** 345–50.

92 Snow AD, Mar H, Nochlin D *et al.* (1990) Early accumulation of heparan sulphate in neurones and in the beta-amyloid protein-containing lesions of Alzheimer's disease and Down's syndrome. *Am J Pathol.* **137:** 1253–70.

93 Iwatsubo T, Mann DMA, Odaka A *et al.* (1995) Amyloid β protein (Aβ) deposition: Aβ42(43) precedes Aβ40 in Down syndrome. *Ann Neurol.* **37:** 294–9.

94 Mann DMA, Iwatsubo T, Fukumoto H *et al.* (1995) Microglial cells and amyloid β protein (Aβ) deposition: association with Aβ_{40}-containing plaques. *Acta Neuropathol.* **90:** 472–7.

95 Mann DMA, Pickering-Brown SM, Siddons MA *et al.* (1995) The extent of amyloid deposition in brain in patients with Down's syndrome does not depend on the apolipoprotein E genotype. *Neurosci Lett.* **196:** 105–8.

96 Lemere CA, Blusztajn JK, Yamaguchi H *et al.* (1996) Sequence of deposition of heterogenous amyloid beta peptides and apo E in Down syndrome: implications for initial events in amyloid plaque formation. *Neurobiol Dis.* **3:** 16–22.

97 Saido TC, Iwatsubo T, Mann DM *et al.* (1995) Dominant and differential deposition of distinct beta-amyloid peptide species, A beta N3 (pE), in senile plaques. *Neuron.* **14:** 457–66.

98 Iwatsubo T, Saido TC, Mann DMA *et al.* (1996) Full-length amyloid-β-(1–42(43)) and amino-terminally modified and truncated amyloid-β-42(43) deposits in diffuse plaques. *Am J Pathol.* **149:** 1823–30.

99 Saido TC, Yamao-Harigaya W, Iwatsubo T *et al.* (1996) Amino- and carboxyl-terminal heterogeneity of β-amyloid peptides deposited in human brain. *Neurosci Lett.* **215:** 173–6.

100 Kuo YM, Emmerling MR, Woods AS *et al.* (1997) Isolation, chemical characterization, and quantitation of A beta-3-pyroglutamyl peptide from neuritic plaques and vascular amyloid deposits. *Biochem Biophys Res Commun.* **237:** 188–91.

101 Russo C, Saido TC, DeBusk LM *et al.* (1997) Heterogeneity of water-soluble amyloid beta-peptide in Alzheimer's disease and Down's syndrome brains. *FEBS Lett.* **409:** 411–16.

102 Russo C, Salis S, Dolcini V *et al.* (2001) Identification of amino-terminally and phosphotyrosine-modified carboxy-terminal fragments of the amyloid precursor protein in Alzheimer's disease and Down's syndrome brain. *Neurobiol Dis.* **8:** 173–80.

103 Mann DMA, Younis N, Stoddard RW *et al.* (1992) The time course of pathological events concerned with plaque formation in Down's syndrome with particular reference to the involvement of microglial cells. *Neurodegeneration.* **1:** 201–15.

104 Szumanska G, Vorbrodt AW, Mandybur TI *et al.* (1987) Lectin histochemistry of plaques and tangles in Alzheimer's disease. *Acta Neuropathol.* **73:** 1–11.

105 Mann DMA, Bonshek RE, Marcyniuk B *et al.* (1988) Saccharides of senile plaques and neurofibrillary tangles in Alzheimer's disease. *Neurosci Lett.* **85:** 277–82.

106 Kida E, Choi-Miura N-M and Wisniewski KE (1995) Deposition of apolipoproteins E and J in senile plaques is topographically determined in both Alzheimer's disease and Down's syndrome brain. *Brain Res.* **685**: 211–16.

107 Wisniewski T and Frangione B (1992) Apolipoprotein E: a pathological chaperone in patients with cerebral and systemic amyloid. *Neurosci Lett.* **135**: 235–8.

108 Schmidt ML, Lee VM-Y, Forman M *et al.* (1997) Monoclonal antibodies to a 100-kd protein reveal abundant Aβ-negative plaques throughout gray matter of Alzheimer's disease brains. *Am J Pathol.* **151**: 69–80.

109 Lemere CA, Grenfell J and Selkoe DJ (1999) The AMY antigen co-occurs with Aβ and follows its deposition in the amyloid plaques of Alzheimer's disease and Down syndrome. *Am J Pathol.* **155**: 29–37.

110 Kowa H, Sakakura T, Matsuura Y *et al.* (2004) Mostly separate distributions of CLAC versus Abeta 40 or Thioflavin S reactivities in senile plaques reveal two distinct subpopulations of beta-amyloid deposits. *Am J Pathol.* **165**: 273–81.

111 Ikeda S-I, Allsop D and Glenner GG (1989) The morphology and distribution of plaque and related deposits in the brains of Alzheimer's disease and control cases: an immunohistochemical study using amyloid β protein antibody. *Lab Invest.* **60**: 113–22.

112 Joachim CL, Morris JH and Selkoe DJ (1989) Diffuse amyloid plaques occur commonly in the cerebellum in Alzheimer's disease. *Am J Pathol.* **135**: 309–19.

113 Ogomori K, Kitamoto T, Tateishi J *et al.* (1989) β protein amyloid is widely distributed in the central nervous system of patients with Alzheimer's disease. *Am J Pathol.* **134**: 243–51.

114 Wisniewski HM, Bancher C, Barcikowska M *et al.* (1989) Spectrum of morphological appearance of amyloid deposits in Alzheimer's disease. *Acta Neuropathol.* **78**: 337–47.

115 Yamaguchi H, Hirai S, Morimatsu M *et al.* (1989) Diffuse type of senile plaque in the cerebellum of Alzheimer-type dementia as detected by β-protein immunostaining. *Acta Neuropathol.* **77**: 314–19.

116 Suenaga T, Hirano A, Llena JF *et al.* (1990) Modified Bielschowsky staining and immunohistochemical studies on striatal plaques in Alzheimer's disease. *Acta Neuropathol.* **80**: 280–6.

117 Mann DMA and Iwatsubo T (1996) Diffuse plaques in the cerebellum and corpus striatum in Down's syndrome contain amyloid β protein (A beta) only in the form of A beta 42(43). *Neurodegeneration.* **5**: 115–20.

118 Teller JK, Russo C, DeBusk LM *et al.* (1996) Presence of soluble amyloid beta-peptide precedes amyloid plaque formation in Down's syndrome. *Nature Med.* **2**: 93–5.

119 Hosoda R, Saido TC, Otvos L *et al.* (1998) Quantification of modified amyloid β peptides in Alzheimer's disease and Down's syndrome brains. *J Neuropathol Exp Neurol.* **57**: 1089–95.

120 Glenner GG and Wong CW (1984) Alzheimer's disease: initial report of the purification and characterization of a novel cerebrovascular amyloid protein. *Biochem Biophys Res Commun.* **120**: 885–90.

121 Glenner GG and Wong CW (1984) Alzheimer's disease and Down's syndrome: sharing a unique cerebrovascular amyloid fibril. *Biochem Biophys Res Commun.* **122**: 1131–5.

122 Joachim CL, Duffy LK, Morris JH *et al.* (1988) Protein chemical and immunocytochemical studies of meningovascular β amyloid protein in Alzheimer's disease and normal ageing. *Brain Res.* **474**: 100–11.

123 Delacourte A and Defossez A (1986) Alzheimer's disease tau proteins, the promoting factors of microtubule assembly, are major components of paired helical filaments. *J Neurol Sci.* **76**: 173–86.

124 Ihara Y, Nukina N, Miura R *et al.* (1986) Phosphorylated tau protein is integrated into paired helical filaments in Alzheimer's disease. *J Biochem. (Tokyo)* **99**: 1807–10.

125 Kosik KS, Joachim CL and Selkoe DJ (1986) Microtubule associated protein tau is a major antigenic component of paired helical filaments in Alzheimer's disease. *Proc Natl Acad Sci USA.* **83:** 4044–8.

126 Wood JG, Mirra SS, Pollock NJ *et al.* (1986) Neurofibrillary tangles of Alzheimer's disease share antigenic determinants with the axonal microtubule associated protein tau. *Proc Natl Acad Sci USA.* **83:** 4040–3.

127 Kosik KS, Orecchio LD, Binder LI *et al.* (1988) Epitopes that span the tau molecule are shared with PHF. *Neuron.* **1:** 817–25.

128 Goedert M, Wischik C, Crowther RA *et al.* (1988) Cloning and sequencing of the cDNA encoding a core protein of the paired helical filament of Alzheimer's disease: identification as the microtubule-associated protein, tau. *Proc Natl Acad Sci USA.* **85:** 4051–5.

129 Wischik C, Novak M, Thagersen HC *et al.* (1988) Isolation of a fragment of tau derived from the core of the paired helical filament of Alzheimer's disease. *Proc Natl Acad Sci USA.* **85:** 4506–10.

130 Mori H, Kondo J and Ihara Y (1987) Ubiquitin is a component of paired helical filament in Alzheimer's disease. *Science.* **235:** 1641–4.

131 Perry G, Friedman R, Shaw G *et al.* (1987) Ubiquitin is detected in neurofibrillary tangles and senile plaque neurites of Alzheimer's disease brains. *Proc Natl Acad Sci USA.* **84:** 3033–6.

132 Lennox G, Lowe JS, Morrell K *et al.* (1988) Ubiquitin is a component of neurofibrillary tangles in a variety of neurodegenerative disorders. *Neurosci Lett.* **94:** 211–17.

133 Lowe J, Blanchard A, Morrell K *et al.* (1988) Ubiquitin is a common factor in intermediate filament inclusion bodies of diverse type in man including those of Parkinson's disease, Pick's disease and Alzheimer's disease, as well as Rosenthal fibres in cerebellar astrocytomas, cytoplasmic bodies in muscle and Mallory bodies in alcoholic liver disease. *J Pathol.* **155:** 9–15.

134 Sparkman DR, Hill SJ and White CL (1990) Paired helical filaments are not major binding sites for WGA and DBA agglutinins in neurofibrillary tangles of Alzheimer's disease. *Acta Neuropathol.* **79:** 640–6.

135 Mann DMA, Prinja D, Davies CA *et al.* (1989) Immunocytochemical profile of neurofibrillary tangles in Down's syndrome patients of different ages. *J Neurol Sci.* **92:** 247–60.

136 Flament S, Delacourte A and Mann DMA (1990) Phosphorylation of tau proteins: a major event during the process of neurofibrillary degeneration. Comparisons between Alzheimer's disease and Down's syndrome. *Brain Res.* **516:** 15–19.

137 Hanger DP, Brion J-P, Gallo J-M *et al.* (1991) Tau in Alzheimer's disease and Down's syndrome is insoluble and abnormally phosphorylated. *Biochem J.* **275:** 99–104.

138 Rohn TT, Head E, Hesse PW *et al.* (2001) Activation of caspase-8 in the Alzheimer disease brain. *Neurobiol Dis.* **8:** 1006–16.

139 Adamec E, Mohan P, Vonsattel JP *et al.* (2002) Calpain activation in neurodegenerative disease: confocal immunofluorescence study with antibodies specifically recognising the active form of calpain 2. *Acta Neuropathol.* **104:** 92–104.

140 Head E, Lott IT, Cribbs DH *et al.* (2002) β-amyloid deposition and neurofibrillary tangle association with caspase activation in Down syndrome. *Neurosci Lett.* **330:** 99–103.

141 Su JH, Kesslak JP, Head E *et al.* (2002) Caspase-cleaved amyloid precursor protein and activated caspase-3 are co-localised in the granules of granulovacuolar degeneration in Alzheimer's disease and Down's syndrome brain. *Acta Neuropathol.* **104:** 1–6.

142 Gibb WRG, Mountjoy CQ, Mann DMA *et al.* (1989) A pathological study of the association between Lewy body disease and Alzheimer disease. *J Neurol Neurosurg Psychiatry.* **52:** 701–8.

143 Raghavan R, Khin-Nu C and Brown A (1993) Detection of Lewy bodies in trisomy 21. *Can J Neurol Sci.* **20:** 48–51.

144 Bodhireddy S, Dickson DW, Mattiace L *et al.* (1994) A case of Down's syndrome with diffuse Lewy body disease and Alzheimer's disease. *Neurology.* **44**: 159–61.

145 Hestnes A, Daniel SE, Lees AJ *et al.* (1996) Down's syndrome and Parkinson's disease. *J Neurol Neurosurg Psychiatry.* **53**: 289.

146 Gibb WRG, Mountjoy CQ, Mann DMA *et al.* (1989) The substantia nigra and ventral tegmental area in Alzheimer's disease and Down's syndrome. *J Neurol Neurosurg Psychiatry.* **52**: 193–200.

147 Lippa CF, Fujiwara H, Mann DMA *et al.* (1998) Lewy bodies contain altered alpha-synuclein in brains of many familial Alzheimer's disease patients with mutations in presenilin and amyloid precursor protein genes. *Am J Pathol.* **153**: 1365–70.

148 Lippa CF, Schmidt ML, Lee VM-Y *et al.* (1999) Antibodies to α-synuclein detect Lewy bodies in many Down syndrome brains with Alzheimer's disease. *Ann Neurol.* **45**: 353–7.

149 Wisniewski KE, Frenchy JH, Rosen JF *et al.* (1982) Basal ganglia calcification (BGC) in Down's syndrome (DS) – another manifestation of premature ageing. *Ann N Y Acad Sci.* **396**: 179–89.

150 Takashima S and Becker LE (1985) Basal ganglia calcification in Down's syndrome. *J Neurol Neurosurg Psychiatry.* **48**: 61–4.

151 Mann DMA (1988) Calcification of the basal ganglia in Down's syndrome and Alzheimer's disease. *Acta Neuropathol.* **76**: 595–8.

152 Colon EJ (1972) The structure of the cerebral cortex in Down's syndrome. *Neuropaediatrics.* **3**: 362–76.

153 Wisniewski KE, Laure-Kamionowska M and Wisniewski HM (1984) Evidence of arrest of neurogenesis and synaptogenesis in brains of patients with Down's syndrome. *NEJM.* **311**: 1187–8.

154 Gandolfi A, Horoupian DS and DeTeresa RM (1981) Pathology of the auditory system in trisomies with morphometric and quantitative study of the ventral cochlear nucleus. *J Neurol Sci.* **51**: 43–50.

155 Casanova MF, Walker LC, Whitehouse PJ *et al.* (1985) Abnormalities of the nucleus basalis in Down's syndrome. *Ann Neurol.* **18**: 310–13.

156 McGeer EG, Norman M, Boyes B *et al.* (1985) Acetylcholine and aromatic amine systems in post-mortem brain of an infant with Down's syndrome. *Exp Neurol.* **87**: 557–60.

157 Marin-Padilla M (1976) Pyramidal cell abnormalities in the motor cortex of a child with Down's syndrome. A Golgi study. *J Comp Neurol.* **167**: 63–82.

158 Suetsuga M and Mehraein P (1980) Spine distribution along the apical dendrite of the pyramidal neurons in Down's syndrome. A quantitative Golgi study. *Acta Neuropathol.* **50**: 207–10.

159 Takashima S, Becker LE, Armstrong DL *et al.* (1981) Abnormal neuronal development in the visual cortex of the human fetus and infant with Down's syndrome. *Brain Res.* **225**: 1–21.

160 Becker LA, Armstrong DL and Chang F (1986) Dendritic atrophy in children with Down's syndrome. *Ann Neurol.* **20**: 520–7.

161 Wisniewski KE and Schmidt-Sidor B (1986) Myelination in Down's syndrome brains (pre- and post-natal maturation) and some clinical–pathological correlations. *Ann Neurol.* **20**: 429–30.

162 Baffico M, Perroni A, Rasore-Quartino A *et al.* (1989) Expression of the human ETS-2 oncogene in normal fetal tissues and in the brain of a fetus with trisomy 21. *Hum Genet.* **83**: 295–6.

163 Greber-Platzer S, Balcz B, Cairns NJ *et al.* (1999) C-fos expression in brain of patients with Down syndrome. *J Neural Transm.* **57**: 75–86.

164 Labudova O, Krapfenbauer K, Moenkmann H *et al.* (1998) Decreased transcription factor junD in brain of patients with Down syndrome. *Neurosci Lett.* **252**: 159–62.

165 Greber-Platzer S, Turhani-Schatzmann D, Cairns NJ *et al.* (1999) The expression of the transcription factor ets-2 in the brains of patients with Down syndrome. Evidence against the overexpression-gene dosage hypothesis. *J Neural Transm.* **57**: 269–82.

166 Kobayashi K, Emson PC, Mountjoy CQ *et al.* (1990) Cerebral cortical calbindin D_{28k} and parvalbumin neurones in Down's syndrome. *Neurosci Lett.* **113**: 17–22.

167 Hyman BT and Mann DMA (1991) Alzheimer-type pathological changes in Down's individuals of various ages. In: K Iqbal, DRC McLachlan, B Winblad and HM Wisniewski (eds) *Alzheimer's Disease: basic mechanisms, diagnosis and therapeutic strategies.* John Wiley & Sons, New York.

168 Teipel SJ, Schapiro MB, Alexander GE *et al.* (2003) Relation of corpus callosum and hippocampal size to age in non-demented adults with Down's syndrome. *Am J Psychiatry.* **160**: 1870–8.

169 Price DL, Whitehouse PJ, Struble RG *et al.* (1982) Alzheimer's disease and Down's syndrome. *Ann N Y Acad Sci.* **396**: 145–64.

170 Marcyniuk B, Mann DMA and Yates PO (1988) Topography of nerve cell loss from the locus caeruleus in middle-aged persons with Down's syndrome. *J Neurol Sci.* **83**: 15–24.

171 German DC, Manaye KF, White CL *et al.* (1992) Disease-specific patterns of locus caeruleus cell loss: Parkinson's disease, Alzheimer's disease and Down's syndrome. *Ann Neurol.* **32**: 667–76.

172 Mann DMA and Yates PO (1986) Neurotransmitter deficits in Alzheimer's disease and in other dementing disorders. *Hum Neurobiol.* **5**: 147–58.

173 Yates CM, Simpson J, Maloney AFJ *et al.* (1980) Alzheimer-like cholinergic deficiency in Down's syndrome. *Lancet.* **ii**: 979.

174 Godridge H, Reynolds GP, Czudek C *et al.* (1987) Alzheimer-like neurotransmitter deficits in adult Down's syndrome brain tissue. *J Neurol Neurosurg Psychiatry.* **50**: 775–8.

175 Yates CN, Ritchie IM, Simpson J *et al.* (1981) Noradrenaline in Alzheimer-type dementia and Down's syndrome. *Lancet.* **ii**: 39–40.

176 Reynolds GP and Godridge H (1985) Alzheimer-like monoamine deficits in adults with Down's syndrome. *Lancet.* **ii**: 1368–9.

177 Yates CM, Simpson J and Gordon A (1986) Regional brain 5-hydroxytryptamine levels are reduced in senile Down's syndrome as in Alzheimer's disease. *Neurosci Lett.* **65**: 189–92.

178 Reynolds GP and Warner CEJ (1988) Amino acid transmitter deficits in adult Down's syndrome brain tissue. *Neurosci Lett.* **94**: 224–7.

179 Simpson MD, Slater P, Cross AJ *et al.* (1989) Reduced D-[^{3}H] aspartate binding in Down's syndrome brains. *Brain Res.* **484**: 273–8.

180 Pierotti AR, Harmar AJ, Simpson J *et al.* (1986) High-molecular-weight forms of somatostatin are reduced in Alzheimer's disease and Down's syndrome. *Neurosci Lett.* **63**: 141–6.

181 Eikelenboom P and Veerhuis R (1996) The role of complement and activated microglia in the pathogenesis of Alzheimer's disease. *Neurobiol Ageing.* **17**: 673–80.

182 Wegiel J, Wisniewski HM, Dziewiatkowski J *et al.* (1996) Differential susceptibility to neurofibrillary pathology among patients with Down syndrome. *Dementia.* **7**: 135–41.

183 Leverenz JB and Raskind MA (1998) Early amyloid deposition in the medial temporal lobe of young Down syndrome patients: a regional quantitative analysis. *Exp Neurol.* **150**: 296–304.

184 Stoltzner SE, Grenfell TJ, Mori C *et al.* (2000) Temporal accrual of complement proteins in amyloid plaques in Down's syndrome with Alzheimer's disease. *Am J Pathol.* **152**: 489–99.

185 Head E, Azizeh BY, Lott IT *et al.* (2001) Complement association with neurones and β-amyloid deposition in the brains of aged individuals with Down syndrome. *Neurobiol Dis.* **8**: 252–65.

186 Shapira R, Austin GE and Mirra SS (1988) Neuritic plaque amyloid in Alzheimer's disease is highly racemized. *J Neurochem.* **50:** 69–74.

187 Fonseca MI, Head E, Velasquez P *et al.* (1999) The presence of isoaspartic acid in β-amyloid plaques indicates plaque age. *Exp Neurol.* **157:** 277–88.

188 Azizeh BY, Head E, Ibrahim MA *et al.* (2000) Molecular dating of senile plaques in the brains of individuals with Down syndrome and in aged dogs. *Exp Neurol.* **163:** 111–22.

189 Chartier-Harlin MC, Crawford F, Houlden H *et al.* (1991) Mutations at codon 717 of the β amyloid precursor protein gene cause Alzheimer's disease. *Nature.* **353:** 84–6.

190 Goate A, Chartier-Harlin MC, Mullan M *et al.* (1991) Segregation of a missense mutation in the amyloid precursor gene with familial Alzheimer's disease. *Nature.* **349:** 704–6.

191 Murrell J, Farlow M, Ghetti B *et al.* (1991) A mutation in the amyloid precursor protein associated with hereditary Alzheimer's disease. *Science.* **254:** 97–9.

192 Naruse S, Igarashi S, Aoki K *et al.* (1991) Mis-sense mutation val → tile in exon 17 of amyloid precursor protein gene in Japanese familial Alzheimer's disease. *Lancet.* **337:** 978–9.

193 Nishimura M, Yu G and St George-Hyslop PH (1999) Biology of presenilins as causative molecules for Alzheimer disease. *Clin Genet.* **55:** 219–25.

194 Scheuner D, Eckman C, Jensen M *et al.* (1996) Secreted amyloid β-protein similar to that in the senile plaques of Alzheimer's disease is increased *in vivo* by the presenilin 1 and 2 and APP mutations linked to familial Alzheimer's disease. *Nature Med.* **2:** 864–9.

195 Mann DMA, Iwatsubo T, Cairns NJ *et al.* (1996) Amyloid β protein (Aβ) deposition in chromosome-14-linked Alzheimer's disease: predominance of A$\beta_{42(43)}$. Ann Neurol. **40:** 149–56.

196 Mann DMA, Iwatsubo T, Ihara Y *et al.* (1996) Predominant deposition of amyloid-$\beta_{42(43)}$ in plaques in cases of Alzheimer's disease and hereditary cerebral hemorrhage associated with mutations in the amyloid precursor protein gene. *Am J Pathol.* **148:** 1257–66.

197 Mann DMA, Iwatsubo T, Nochlin D *et al.* (1997) Amyloid (Aβ) protein deposition in chromosome-1-linked Alzheimer's disease – the Volga German kindreds. *Ann Neurol.* **41:** 52–7.

198 Mann DMA, Pickering-Brown SM, Takeuchi A *et al.* (2001) Amyloid angiopathy and variability in amyloid β (Aβ) deposition is determined by mutation position in presenilin-1-linked Alzheimer's disease. *Am J Pathol.* **158:** 1865–75.

199 Kang J, Lemaire H-G, Unterbeck A *et al.* (1987) The precursor of Alzheimer's disease amyloid A4 protein resembles a cell-surface receptor. *Nature.* **325:** 733–6.

200 Neve RL, Finch CE and Dawes LR (1988) Expression of the Alzheimer amyloid precursor gene transcripts in human brain. *Neuron.* **1:** 669–77.

201 Oyama F, Cairns NJ, Shimada H *et al.* (1994) Down's syndrome: upregulation of beta-amyloid precursor protein and tau mRNAs and their defective coordination. *J Neurochem.* **62:** 1062–6.

202 Rowe IF, Ridler MAC and Gibberd FB (1989) Presenile dementia associated with mosaic trisomy 21 in a patient with a Down's syndrome child. *Lancet.* **2:** 229.

203 Schapiro MB, Kumar A, White B *et al.* (1989) Alzheimer's disease (AD) in mosaic/translocation Down's syndrome (DS) without mental retardation. *Neurology.* **39 (Suppl. 1):** 169.

204 Sinet PM, Michelson AM, Bazin A *et al.* (1975) Increase in glutathione peroxidase activity in erythrocytes from trisomy 21 subjects. *Biochem Biophys Res Commun.* **67:** 910–15.

205 Brooksbank BW and Balazs R (1984) Superoxide dismutase, glutathione peroxidase and lipoperoxidation in Down's syndrome fetal brain. *Brain Res.* **318:** 37–44.

206 Anneren G and Epstein CJ (1987) Lipid peroxidation and superoxide dismutase-1 and glutathione peroxidase activities in trisomy 16 fetal mice and human trisomy 21 fibroblasts. *Pediatr Res.* **21:** 88–92.

207 Gulesserian T, Fountoulakis M, Seidl R *et al.* (2001) Superoxide dismutase SOD1, encoded on chromosome 21, but not SOD2 is overexpressed in the brains of patients with Down syndrome. *J Invest Med.* **49:** 41–6.

208 Griffin WST, Stanley LC, Ling C *et al.* (1989) Brain interleukin 1 and S100 immunoreactivity are elevated in Down's syndrome and Alzheimer's disease. *Proc Natl Acad Sci USA.* **86:** 7611–15.

209 Mito T and Becker LE (1993) Developmental changes of S-100 protein and glial fibrillary acidic protein in the brain in Down syndrome. *Exp Neurol.* **120:** 170–6.

210 Griffin WST, Sheng JG, McKenzie JE *et al.* (1998) Lifelong overexpression of S100β in Down's syndrome: implications for Alzheimer pathogenesis. *Neurobiol Ageing.* **19:** 401–5.

211 Li YK, Wong JZ, Sheng JG *et al.* (1998) S100β increases β-amyloid precursor protein and its encoding mRNA in rat neuronal cultures. *J Neurochem.* **71:** 1421–8.

212 Royston MC, McKenzie JE, Gentleman SM *et al.* (1999) Overexpression of S100β in Down's syndrome: correlation with patient age and β-amyloid deposition. *Neuropathol Appl Neurobiol.* **25:** 387–93.

213 Acquati F, Accarino M, Nucci C *et al.* (2000) The gene encoding DRAP (BACE2), a glycosylated transmembrane protein of the aspartic protease family, maps to the down critical region. *FEBS Lett.* **468:** 59–64.

214 Motonaga K, Itoh M, Becker LE *et al.* (2002) Elevated expression of beta-site amyloid precursor protein cleaving enzyme 2 in brains of patients with Down syndrome. *Neurosci Lett.* **326:** 64–6.

215 Wolvetang EW, Bradfield OM, Tymms M *et al.* (2003) The chromosome 21 transcription factor ETS2 transactivates the β-APP promoter: implications for Down syndrome. *Biochim Biophys Acta.* **1626:** 105–10.

216 Corder EH, Saunders AM, Strittmatter WJ *et al.* (1993) Gene dose of apolipoprotein E type 4 allele and the risk of Alzheimer's disease in late-onset families. *Science.* **261:** 921–3.

217 Saunders AM, Schmader K and Breitner J (1993) Apolipoprotein E e4 allele distributions in late-onset Alzheimer's disease and in other amyloid-forming diseases. *Lancet.* **342:** 710–11.

218 Hardy J, Crook R, Perry R *et al.* (1994) Apo E genotype and Down's syndrome. *Lancet.* **343:** 979–80.

219 Hyman BT, West HL, Rebeck GW *et al.* (1995) Neuropathological changes in Down's syndrome hippocampal formation: effect of age and apolipoprotein E genotype. *Arch Neurol.* **52:** 373–8.

220 Martins RN, Clarnette R, Fisher C *et al.* (1995) Apo E genotypes in Australia: roles in early and late onset Alzheimer's disease and Down's syndrome. *Neuroreport.* **6:** 1513–16.

221 Wisniewski T, Morelli L, Wegiel J *et al.* (1995) The influence of apolipoprotein E isotypes on Alzheimer's disease pathology in 40 cases of Down's syndrome. *Ann Neurol.* **37:** 136–8.

222 Van Gool WA, Evenhuis HM and Van Duijn CM (1995) A case–control study of apolipoprotein E genotypes in Alzheimer's disease associated with Down's syndrome. *Ann Neurol.* **38:** 225–30.

223 Avramopoulos D, Mikkelsen M, Vassilopoulos D *et al.* (1996) Apolipoprotein E allele distribution in parents of Down's syndrome children. *Lancet.* **347:** 862–5.

224 Cosgrave M, Tyrrell J, Dreja H *et al.* (1996) Lower frequency of apolipoprotein E4 allele in an 'elderly' Down's syndrome population. *Biol Psychiatry.* **40:** 811–13.

225 Holder JL, Habbak RA, Pearlson GD *et al.* (1996) Reduced survival of apolipoprotein E4 homozygotes in Down's syndrome. *Neuroreport.* **7:** 2455–6.

226 Del Bo R, Comi GP, Bresolin N *et al.* (1997) The apolipoprotein E ϵ4 allele causes a faster decline of cognitive performances in Down's syndrome subjects. *J Neurol Sci.* **145:** 87–91.

227 Prasher VP, Chowdhury TA, Rowe BR *et al.* (1997) Apo E genotype and Alzheimer's disease in adults with Down syndrome: meta-analysis. *Am J Ment Retard.* **102:** 103–10.

228 Talbot C, Lendon C, Craddock N *et al.* (1994) Protection against Alzheimer's disease with Apo E e2. *Lancet.* **343:** 1432–3.

229 Gearing M, Mori H and Mirra SS (1996) Aβ peptide length and apolipoprotein E genotype in Alzheimer's disease. *Ann Neurol.* **39:** 395–9.

230 Mann DMA, Iwatsubo T, Pickering-Brown SM *et al.* (1997) Preferential deposition of amyloid β protein (Aβ) in the form Aβ_{40} in Alzheimer's disease is associated with a gene dosage effect of the apolipoprotein E E4 allele. *Neurosci Lett.* **221:** 81–4.

231 Wragg M, Hutton M, Talbot C *et al.* (1996) Genetic association between intronic polymorphism in the presenilin-1 gene and late-onset Alzheimer's disease. *Lancet.* **347:** 509–12.

232 Kamboh M, Sanghera D, Ferrell R *et al.* (1995) Apo E ϵ4-associated Alzheimer's disease risk is modified by α1 antichymotrypsin polymorphism. *Nat Genet.* **10:** 486–8.

233 Tyrrell J, Cosgrave M, McPherson J *et al.* (1999) Presenilin 1 and α-1-antichymotrypsin polymorphisms in Down syndrome: no effect on the presence of dementia. *Am J Med Genet.* **88:** 616–20.

Chapter 3

Genetics, Alzheimer's disease and Down syndrome

Nicole Schupf

Introduction

Ageing of adults with Down syndrome (DS) has recently become an issue of great concern because of the high risk of Alzheimer's disease (AD) in this rapidly growing population. Virtually all adults with DS over 35 to 40 years of age exhibit many of the key features of AD neuropathology, and many of these individuals will develop dementia by the time they reach 60 to 70 years of age. Alzheimer's disease is the commonest cause of dementia among older people, and affects parts of the brain that control thought, memory and language abilities, resulting in progressive decline. This decline eventually leads to the complete loss of ability to perform daily activities. Three neuropathological findings are characteristic of AD:

1 neuritic plaques, consisting of extracellular deposits of amyloid β-peptide (Aβ) surrounded by degenerating nerve terminals
2 neurofibrillary tangles, consisting of abnormal filaments containing the protein tau within neurons
3 loss of brain cells and brain mass.

A number of factors have been found to be related to increased risk of dementia in Alzheimer's disease (DAD) in addition to age. A family history of DAD is one well-established risk factor for DAD, pointing to the importance of genetic susceptibility. Other less well-established risk factors include level of education, hormonal status, cardiovascular status and cerebrovascular disease, inflammatory processes, oxidative stress and head injury.

A common pathway for both genetic and environmental risk factors may involve contributions to increased accumulation and deposition of Aβ in neuritic plaques. Individuals with DS are at high risk of this pathology at least in part because of triplication and overexpression of the gene, located on chromosome 21, that codes for beta-amyloid precursor protein (APP), from which the Aβs are derived. This chapter will review the influence of genetic factors on risk of DAD among adults with DS. It will discuss genetic factors that may increase Aβ deposition, genes located on chromosome 21 that are overexpressed and implicated in AD pathogenesis, and factors associated with accelerated ageing and early mortality in individuals with DS.

The amyloid cascade hypothesis

Several lines of evidence suggest that deposition of Aβ, specifically Aβ1–42, is a primary event in the pathogenesis of AD.[1] Aβ1–40 and Aβ1–42, the two major species of Aβ, are generated from a larger membrane-bound protein, APP, through cleavage by specific enzymes, namely β- and γ-secretases (*see* Figure 3.1). In addition, α-secretase cleaves the APP in the middle of the Aβ segment, producing soluble APP and a fragment called p3. Because processing by α-secretase precludes the production of Aβ1–42 and Aβ1–40 peptides, it does not contribute to the formation of neuritic plaques.[2]

Brain and cerebrospinal fluid levels of Aβ1–42 increase early in the development of AD, and are strongly correlated with cognitive decline.[3–5] Mayeux and colleagues found that plasma levels of Aβ1–42 are higher in non-demented elderly individuals who subsequently develop DAD than in those who remain free of dementia.[6,7] Thus risk factors may influence the likelihood of development of DAD by increasing production of Aβ or by reduced clearance and excess deposition of Aβ.

Genetic factors appear to influence the risk of developing DAD through a common pathway resulting in increased production or deposition of Aβ1–42.[8]

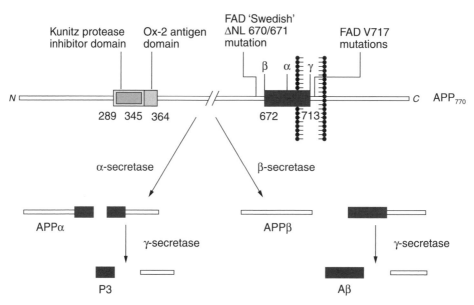

Figure 3.1 APP and its proteolytic products. APP can undergo proteolytic processing via two pathways. Cleavage by α-secretase occurs within the Aβ domain and generates the large soluble N-terminal APPa and a non-amyloidogenic C-terminal fragment. Further proteolysis of this fragment by γ-secretase generates the non-amyloidogenic peptide p3. Alternatively, cleavage of APP by β-secretase occurs at the beginning of the Aβ domain and generates a shorter soluble N-terminus, APPβ, as well as an amyloid-ogenic C-terminal fragment (C99). Further cleavage of this C-terminal fragment by γ-secretase generates Aβ. Cleavage by γ-secretases or multiple γ-secretases can result in C-terminal heterogeneity of Aβ to generate Aβ1–40 and Aβ1–42. Reprinted from Wilson C, Doms RM and Lee VM-Y (1999) Intracellular APP processing and Aβ production in Alzheimer's disease. *J Neuropathol Exp Neurol.* **58**: 787–94, with the permission of Lippincott, Williams & Wilkins, Philadelphia.

To date, four genes have been associated with the development of early-onset (below 60 years of age) or late-onset (above 60 years) DAD. These include three genes associated with very rare cases of early-onset familial forms of AD (FAD) which are transmitted as an autosomal-dominant disease, with almost all mutation carriers being affected.[8-12] These FAD early-onset genes include mutations in the genes for APP, located on chromosome 21, and the presenilins (PS1, located on chromosome 14, and PS2, located on chromosome 1). Together these three genes account for approximately 50% of early-onset DAD (up to 60 years of age) but less than 2% of all cases of DAD. The majority of early-onset DAD is due to mutations in the PS1 gene.[13] There are multiple mutation sites in the genes for APP and in presenilins,[14-16] and these mutations appear to interfere with the normal APP processing pathway and result in an increase in the production of neurotoxic $A\beta1$–42.[8,17] Consistent with the familial aggregation of FAD, plasma $A\beta$ levels are elevated in family members with mutations in PS1 or in the gene for APP.[16]

The fourth gene associated with an increased risk of DAD, located on chromosome 19, is apolipoprotein E (ApoE). Apolipoprotein E has three common alleles, $\epsilon2$, $\epsilon3$ and $\epsilon4$, giving rise to six genotypes. These three variants are found in all populations.[18] The presence of the ApoE $\epsilon4$ allele has been associated with increased risk of developing the more common late-onset DAD. The presence of an ApoE $\epsilon4$ allele accounts for approximately 30% of the risk in late-onset DAD.[13] In numerous cross-sectional and case–control studies, the presence of the ApoE $\epsilon4$ allele has been linked to earlier onset of DAD,[19-23] and greater accumulation of $A\beta$ neuritic plaques, even in non-demented elderly individuals.[24,25] Age at onset decreases and risk of DAD increases with increasing number of ApoE $\epsilon4$ alleles.[19-23]

Although the ApoE $\epsilon4$ allele is a major genetic susceptibility factor for late-onset DAD, other genes that influence age at onset or risk of developing the disease are likely to be discovered. For example, genome-wide linkage analysis in extended families with multiple affected members, and linkage disequilibrium studies in late-onset DAD, have identified several candidate loci for genes for late-onset DAD on a number of chromosomes[8,13] (*see* Table 3.1). Because these genes

Table 3.1 Genes and gene loci associated with Alzheimer's disease

Chromosome	Type	Age at onset (years)	Cases (%)	Gene
21	Autosomal dominant	45–65	<1%	APP
14	Autosomal dominant	28–62	<1%	PS1
1	Autosomal dominant	45–65	<1%	PS2
19	Risk factor	>60	30%	ApoE $\epsilon4$
12	Risk factor	>70	?	$?\alpha2M$ $?LRP$-1
10	Risk factor	>60	?	?IDE

$\alpha2M$ = alpha-2-macroglobulin; LRP-1 = low density lipoprotein-related protein 1; IDE = insulin-degrading enzyme have not been definitively identified, and their role in dementia in DS has yet to be determined, they will not be considered further here.

Down syndrome and Alzheimer's disease

Middle-aged and older adults with DS show age-related changes in health and functional capacity that suggest premature or accelerated ageing.[26] Increased risk of DAD is a major concern. Adults with DS have high levels of Aβ in the brain by the age of 40 years, and their risk of dementia increases around 20 years earlier than it does in their peers without DS.[27,28] The neuropathological manifestations of AD in DS have been attributed at least in part to triplication and overexpression of the gene for APP located on chromosome 21,[29] leading to an increased substrate for production of Aβ.[30] However, clinical and epidemiological studies have shown that age-specific rates of DAD among adults with DS are lower than would be expected given the extensive amyloid and neurofibrillary pathology that is found at autopsy in this population.[28,31] Studies have shown that the average age of onset of dementia ranges from 38 to 70 years, with most cases occurring between 50 and 55 years of age.[28,30,32–41] Even at ages associated with extensive neuropathology, a substantial proportion of elderly people with DS remain functionally unimpaired.

Numerous studies have shown that diffuse plaques, the most prevalent 'Alzheimer-type' neuropathology seen in individuals with DS before the age of 50 years, are not associated with dementia.[42] Diffuse plaques contain non-fibrillar amyloid, appear at younger ages than do neuritic plaques, are not associated with neuronal degeneration, and do not appear to affect the structure and function of neurons.[42] In contrast, increases in the numbers of neuritic plaques, which contain substantial amounts of fibrillar Aβ, are observed in adults with DS predominantly after 50 years of age, and are associated with neuronal degeneration and eventual loss of function.[42] Thus the clinical manifestations of AD in DS are closely associated with the development of plaques containing fibrillar amyloid.[30] Although triplication of the gene for APP may act to increase deposition of Aβ in diffuse plaques in adults with DS, additional genetic and environmental factors which modify the rate and degree of Aβ fibrillisation may be important determinants of age at onset and risk of developing dementia in DS.[30]

Compared with individuals without DS, adults with DS are also at increased risk of developing DAD through accelerated or premature ageing and through triplication and overexpression of genes in addition to APP that are located on chromosome 21. Some of these genes have been implicated in the pathogenesis of AD. They include beta-site amyloid precursor protein-cleaving enzyme (BACE-2), superoxide dismutase-1 (SOD1) and the astrocyte-derived neurotrophic factor S-100β. Gene–gene and gene–environment interactions may also play a role in modifying age at onset and clinical expression of dementia in DS, and contribute to the wide range of age at onset. The remainder of this chapter will review the genetic factors associated with increased risk of developing DAD in DS and the genetic factors associated with individual differences in age at onset, including the following:

1 overexpression of genes located on chromosome 21 that may contribute to the overall increased risk of DAD in adults with DS (APP, BACE-2 and S-100β) (the relationship with SOD1 is covered in depth in Chapter 5)

2 polymorphisms in the genes for APP, presenilins and ApoE that may contribute to individual differences in risk within the DS population
3 factors associated with accelerated ageing.

Dementia associated with overexpression of genes on chromosome 21

Beta amyloid peptides

As noted above, there is strong evidence that altered metabolism of Aβ peptides and amyloid deposition in neuritic plaques cause AD by triggering a complex pathological cascade that destroys neural networks and produces dementia.

Although both Aβ1–42 and Aβ1–40 can be formed when APP is cleaved, deposition of Aβ1–42 in extracellular spaces, rather than deposition of Aβ1–40, appears to be the critical initial step in the pathogenesis of AD. As described above, mutations in the gene for APP and in presenilin (PS1 and PS2) genes are associated with early-onset familial DAD and with a selective increase in Aβ1–42.[2,14–16,43,44] Aβ1–42 aggregates more rapidly and is deposited earlier in AD plaques than Aβ1–40,[1] so that elevated brain and cerebrospinal fluid levels of Aβ1–42 are among the earliest markers of incipient AD.[3–5] In both cerebrospinal fluid and plasma, Aβ1–42 levels decline with disease progression.[4–6] Thus in prevalent cases of DAD, Aβ1–42 levels may be lower or higher than in non-demented controls, depending upon the stage of the disease process. The decrease in cerebrospinal fluid and plasma Aβ1–42 levels with disease progression has been attributed to the removal of circulating Aβ and its deposition in neuritic plaques. These changes in Aβ levels with disease progression complicate epidemiological investigation, as careful matching of study participants by disease duration and stage is required in order to detect effects or compare results across studies, and this can be difficult to achieve.

Ertekin-Taner and colleagues have suggested that individual differences in Aβ levels are influenced by genetic factors.[45] They estimated the heritability of plasma Aβ1–42 and Aβ1–40 levels in families with late-onset DAD to be as high as 73% and 54% for plasma Aβ1–42 and Aβ1–40 levels, respectively. This association may be influenced by a gene (or genes) on chromosome 10.[46–48] The investigators suggest that the high degree of heritability and the significant elevation of Aβ in late-onset DAD pedigrees indicate that genetic determinants may lead to elevated Aβ levels and increase the risk of developing DAD.[45]

In adults with DS, as in adults in the general population with DAD, deposition of Aβ1–42 precedes the appearance of Aβ1–40 in plaques.[49] Aβ1–42 has been observed to be the predominant peptide in the brains of young individuals (under 50 years of age) with DS, while Aβ1–40 deposits were observed only a decade or more later.[50] Even in older adults with DS (over 50 years of age), plaques containing Aβ1–42 are more abundant than those containing Aβ1–40. These findings support the hypothesis that triplication and overexpression of APP represent a critical step in the development of AD in adults with DS. This hypothesis is supported by an interesting case presented by Prasher and colleagues[51] of a 78-year-old woman with partial trisomy 21, namely 46,XX,rec(21)dup q, inv(21)(p12q22.1). Although her appearance was not typical, her medical history included several of the common age-related medical conditions that are characteristic of an elderly person with DS, including hypothyroidism, cataracts, hypotonia and hearing impairment. Analysis of gene sequences on chromosome 21 showed that her partial trisomy excluded the region containing the gene for APP, which was present in only two copies. There was no evidence of a decline in cognitive or adaptive competence for the five years preceding her death from pneumonia, and no evidence of AD was found on neuropathological assessment. These findings support the hypothesis that over-expression of APP and excess Aβ levels are necessary for the early onset of DAD in adults with DS.[30,51]

Compared with age-matched controls from the general population, blood levels of both Aβ1–42 and Aβ1–40 are increased in adults with DS.[52–55] Mehta and colleagues found that plasma Aβ1–42 levels in young individuals with DS and controls were similar. However, Aβ1–42 levels were higher in older individuals with DS than in younger individuals with DS or controls. They concluded that in older adults with DS, Aβ1–42 is selectively increased in plasma concurrently with the development of AD neuropathology.[56] Schupf and colleagues compared plasma Aβ1–42 and Aβ1–40 levels in demented and non-demented adults with DS with the plasma levels in non-demented adults from the general population.[54] Aβ1–42 and Aβ1–40 levels were significantly higher in adults with DS than in controls from the general population ($P = 0.0001$), and were highest in demented adults with DS. Furthermore, the presence of the ApoE ϵ4 allele was associated with increased plasma levels of Aβ1–42, but not of Aβ1–40, in both non-demented and demented adults (*see* Figure 3.2). The effect of the ApoE ϵ4 allele on Aβ1–42 levels may be related to acceleration of the rate of amyloid fibril formation,[57] or to reduced clearance of Aβ.[58]

In contrast, Cavani and colleagues did not find an association between plasma levels of Aβ1–42 and the ApoE genotype.[52] They concluded that the accumulation and clearance of plasma and cerebral Aβ are regulated by different and independent factors. Tokuda and colleagues examined the relationship between Aβ peptides and dementia but, unlike Schupf and colleagues, they failed to find a difference in Aβ levels between demented and non-demented adults with DS.[55] Differences in subject recruitment, case definition and duration of dementia may account for the different findings in these studies. The cases of DAD in the study by Schupf and colleagues were of relatively recent onset, but if the cases examined by Tokuda and colleagues were of longer duration, then a decrease in Aβ1–42 levels would be expected with disease progression, and this could account for the failure to find a difference between demented and non-demented individuals in that study. Tapiola and colleagues observed an age-dependent decrease in cerebrospinal fluid levels of Aβ1–42 that was independent of the presence of the ApoE genotype and an age-related increase in cerebrospinal fluid levels of tau protein.[59] These results are consistent with findings in cerebrospinal fluid from patients with DAD in the general population,[60] suggesting that there is removal of circulating Aβ through plaque formation in the brain.

In summary, these findings support the hypothesis that individual differences in Aβ processing, distinct from overexpression of APP per se, may represent an initial step in the pathogenesis of AD in individuals with and without DS. Heritable individual differences in Aβ levels associated with genetic variants that have yet to be determined may be related to age at onset of dementia and

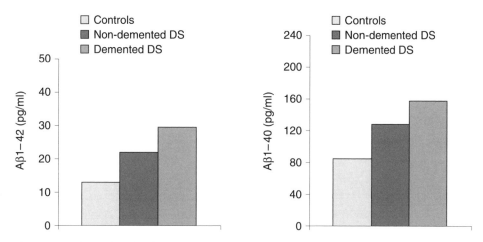

Figure 3.2 Plasma levels of Aβ1–42 and Aβ1–40 in demented and non-demented adults with Down syndrome. Reprinted from Schupf N, Patel B, Silverman W *et al.* (2001) Elevated plasma amyloid β-peptide 1–42 and onset of dementia in Down syndrome. *Neurosci Lett.* **301**: 199–203, with the permission of Elsevier Publishers, Oxford. (Modified)

rate of disease progression. It is tempting to consider whether plasma levels of Aβ1–42 might serve as a biomarker for dementia risk in adults with DS, facilitating early diagnosis or intervention to delay or prevent onset. However, examination of data at an individual level from all studies reveals considerable overlap in plasma levels of both Aβ1–42 and Aβ1–40 between demented and non-demented adults. In addition, the relationship between plasma and brain levels of Aβ is not yet fully understood. In part, the evaluation of plasma Aβ levels as biomarkers for AD is limited by the lack of longitudinal studies in which established non-demented individuals are followed to the point of onset of dementia. This is an especially important point, given that plasma levels of Aβ1–42 are expected first to increase and then to decline with disease onset and progression.

BACE

Factors that influence the processing of Aβ may also contribute to the higher levels of Aβ in the brains of older adults with DS. As outlined above, Aβ is generated from full-length APP by cleavage secretases. β-Secretase cleaves full-length APP, producing soluble APP and a C-terminal fragment with Aβ at its amino end. γ-Secretase then cleaves the C-terminal fragment at its carboxyl end, releasing Aβ (*see* Figure 3.1). BACE, a transmembrane protease, has been identified as β-secretase. A homologue of BACE, BACE-2, is located on chromosome 21.[61] As would be expected with triplication of the gene for BACE-2, higher BACE-2 protein levels have been found to be associated with DS.[61] In a neuropathological study of BACE-2 activity, changes in the expression of BACE-2 were investigated immunohistochemically in the frontal cortex of 13 individuals with DS, aged from 27 weeks to 37 years.[62] Immunoreactivity for

BACE-2 was detected in elderly brains with DS that had AD neuropathology, but was not detected in brains without AD neuropathology or in control brains without DS of any age.[62] Thus activity of this protease may contribute to plaque formation in addition to the increased substrate for $A\beta$ formation that results from overexpression of APP.[61,63]

S-100β protein

The S-100β gene is located on chromosome 21 and is overexpressed in association with triplication of chromosome 21. This gene codes for a calcium-binding protein which is produced and secreted by astrocytes in the central and peripheral nervous system.[64,65] S-100β promotes neuron survival and differentiation, neurite extension, synaptogenesis and programmed cell death (apoptosis).[64,65]

The neuritic plaques associated with AD contain dystrophic neuritis, and it has been suggested that the role of S-100β as a neurite extension factor may contribute to the overgrowth of neurites that is characteristic of neuritic plaques.[64,66–69] Tissue levels of S-100β have been found to be elevated by two- to threefold in the brains of individuals with AD without DS compared with non-demented control brains, and the number of S-100β-containing astrocytes was highly correlated with the number of neuritic plaques.[69,70] These findings suggest that overexpression of S-100β may be implicated in the induction of dystrophic neurites in amyloid deposits in AD.[68]

In individuals with DS, triplication and overexpression of the S-100β gene may affect a number of processes related to development, rate of ageing and risk for DAD. There is an approximately twofold lifelong overexpression of S-100β in DS,[66,69] and overexpression of S-100β is observed in plasma as well as in brain. Several investigators have suggested that this overexpression of S-100β is associated with the dendritic and other developmental neuronal abnormalities that are characteristic of DS.[65,66,71–73] Early in development there is an accelerated pace of dendritic maturation with a relatively expanded dendritic tree.[71] However, during the first year of life dendrites appear to stop growing in the brains of individuals with DS and become atrophic relative to control neurons.[71,72,74] These changes may contribute to the ID that is characteristic of individuals with DS, as well as to their increased risk of developing DAD.[71,72,74,75] Transgenic mice produced by insertion of human S-100β genes show similar patterns of developmental neuronal abnormalities and impaired performance on learning tasks.[65,73,76,77]

S-100β overexpression may influence the risk of DAD by a number of pathways in addition to neurite overgrowth. In laboratory studies, S-100β increased levels of APP in primary cultures from rat neuronal cortex,[67] which may influence the development of amyloid plaques and increase the risk for DAD. S-100β may also promote the overexpression of interleukin-1 (IL-1), an inflammatory cytokine, as well as that of APP.[74] IL-1 in turn induces the expression of both S-100β and APP in DS,[66,74] and this pathway might exacerbate the neurotoxic effects.

Royston and colleagues[78] examined the cerebral cortical load of S-100β in 18 individuals with DS aged 13–65 years. They found a high correlation between both S-100β-staining astrocytes and age ($r = 0.6$), and an increase in the ratio of activated to non-activated astrocytes with increasing overall S-100β load. They suggested that there is a higher relative proportion of activated astrocytes with increasing age, perhaps reflecting increasing amyloid burden.[78] A high correlation was also found between S-100β expression and cerebral cortical Aβ deposition (r = 0.77), consistent with a role of S-100β in the induction of APP expression.[67,78] Because of the small sample size, it was not possible to examine the relationship between S-100β expression and Aβ load in age-matched samples of demented and non-demented individuals. When it can be done, this type of analysis should reveal whether there are individual differences in S-100β expression among adults with DS that are related to the development of dementia.

These initial studies suggest that S-100β activity may have an important influence on both the rate of ageing and the risk of dementia in adults with DS. Almost all studies have been conducted on brain tissue at autopsy. Since S-100β protein levels are elevated in plasma as well as in brain tissue in individuals with DS, larger-scale epidemiological studies should be possible, and could provide a means of examining whether individual differences in plasma S-100β levels modulate Aβ peptide levels and are associated with age at onset of DAD.

Polymorphisms in presenilins, APP and ApoE

While an overall increased risk of developing DAD may be related to over-expression of genes located on chromosome 21, variation in risk for DAD may also be influenced by genes that are not localised to chromosome 21. As noted above, mutations in presenilins, as well as in APP, are associated with early-onset familial forms of DAD.[8–12] These mutations are extremely rare and would not be expected to contribute to risk of DAD in DS. However, normal variants in regulatory sequences in presenilins and APP might influence age at onset and risk of late-onset DAD by increasing Aβ production through changing patterns of APP splicing or influencing APP promoter activity.[79,80]

Only a few studies have examined the relationship between polymorphisms in these genes and DAD, and the findings have been inconsistent. In some cases the samples have been too young to provide evidence of a strong relationship to dementia.[81] Tyrrell and colleagues examined a common polymorphism in PS1 in adults with DS, and found no significant differences in PS1 1–allele frequencies between demented and age-matched non-demented adults with DS.[82]

In a cross-sectional study, a relationship between a tetranucleotide repeat variant in a coding region of the APP gene (APP6) and age at onset of dementia in 105 adults with DS was recently reported.[80] Mean age at onset of dementia in the total sample was 50.9 years. Age at onset of dementia was 13 years later, on average, in individuals with fewer than three repeat APP6 alleles (mean age at onset 53.8 years) compared with individuals with three or more APP6 alleles (mean age at onset 40.0 years).[80] The investigators suggest that the effect of repeat length on age at onset may be mediated through polymorphic variations in the promoter region of APP, leading to altered basal transcription levels of Aβ.[79,80,83] However, the very early age of onset in this sample is unusual, and raises concern about the diagnostic criteria. Although the mean age at onset was 50.9 years, 15% of the sample developed dementia before the age of 45 years. Most studies of the incidence and prevalence of dementia in adults with DS report that approximately 5% of adults with DS aged 40–45 years would be expected to have dementia.[33,35,36,40,84,85] Re-examination and replication of this interesting finding in future studies should be strongly encouraged.

The major genetic susceptibility factor for late-onset DAD is the ε4 allele of the ApoE gene. ApoE plays a central role in plasma lipoprotein metabolism and lipid transport within tissues,[86] and is a major constituent of very-low-density lipoprotein (VLDL).[87] As noted above, ApoE is polymorphic in all populations,[18] with three common alleles, ε2, ε3 and ε4, resulting in six genotypes. The ε3 allele is the most frequent one, and the distribution of ApoE alleles is similar among individuals with and without DS (ε2, 7.5%; ε3, 78.9%; ε4, 13.6%).[88] The ApoE ε4 allele has been associated with higher levels of total and low-density-lipoprotein (LDL) cholesterol and increased risk of cardiovascular disease,[87] increased Aβ deposition and earlier onset of DAD.[19–25]

ApoE genotype has also been associated with longevity. In a group of French centenarians, the relative frequency of the ApoE ε2 allele was elevated and that of the ε4 frequency was lowered compared with a younger group, which suggests that the ε2 allele enhanced longevity whereas the ε4 allele contributed to relatively early mortality.[89] Similar elevated ε2 allele frequencies were observed in Japanese and Finnish centenarians.[90–91] However, in other populations the frequency of the ε2 allele was similar in older and younger cohorts, and the frequency of the ε4 allele was not consistently lower in the older cohort.[87,92–95] The presence of the ApoE ε2 allele has been associated with a delay in onset of DAD or even protection against DAD in most studies.[96,97]

Among adults with DS, all studies have consistently found that the presence of the ApoE ε2 allele contributed to increased longevity and reduced risk of dementia.[30,35,88,98–109] Several studies have reported reduced frequencies of the ApoE ε4 allele in 'elderly' groups of individuals with DS, suggesting that the ε4 allele may be associated with early mortality, either in association with dementia or independent of the presence of dementia.[98,110] In contrast, a meta-analysis of the frequency of ε4 homozygotes (ApoE 4/4 genotype) among 538 adults with DS from 11 studies found only the number of ε4 homozygotes that would be expected based on frequencies in the general population.[111] The authors suggested that ε4 homozygosity was not associated with mortality before adulthood in DS.[111] However, the meta-analysis was based on studies that included a high proportion of relatively young adults (under 50 years of age) with DS, and the analysis was not stratified by age group.[111] Thus the role of the ApoE ε4 allele in the early mortality observed among adults with DS over the age of 40 or 50 years is still uncertain, and larger samples of the 'oldest old' with DS (e.g. those over 65 years) will be required in order to resolve this issue.

In neuropathological studies of adults with DS, Hyman and colleagues found that adults with DS with an ApoE ε4 allele had greater deposition of Aβ than those without the ε4 allele.[24] However, the impact of the ε4 allele on risk for dementia has been more difficult to demonstrate than the protective effects of the ε2 allele. This is likely to be due to the fact that the ε4 allele is relatively uncommon, and substantial samples of older individuals are required in order to detect an effect in a population where the rate of dementia is already high. Small sample sizes and, importantly, failure to consider differences in the age at onset of dementia among individuals with and without an ε4 allele may account for some of the negative findings. Since the effect of the ε4 allele is not observed until midlife, inclusion of sufficient numbers of adults over 50 years of age and analysis using survival methods (that can adjust for age and number of years of follow-up) are important methodological considerations.[30]

When survival methods have been used, the presence of the ε4 allele was associated with earlier onset of dementia and a greater decline in adaptive behaviour for adults with DS.[88] Compared with individuals with the ApoE 3/3 genotype, adults with DS with an ε4 allele were almost five times as likely to develop dementia by the age of 65 years (odds ratio = 4.7), while no one with an ε2 allele developed dementia. Among affected individuals, mean age at onset of dementia was 53.3 years for those with the ε4 allele and 58.0 years for those with the 3/3 genotype. Similar findings have been reported by Lai and colleagues.[35] In their study the cumulative incidence of dementia by the age of 65 years was 55% for those with the ApoE 2/3 genotype, 88% for those with the ApoE 3/3 genotype and 100% for those with any ε4 allele.[35] The effect of the ε4 allele was stronger at younger ages, consistent with findings from studies in the general population that the effect of the ε4 allele is to accelerate onset of DAD.[19,112] The cumulative incidence up to age 55 years was 0.71 among individuals with an ε4 allele and 0.40 among those with the ApoE 3/3 genotype. The investigators suggested that the ε4 effect in their study might have been attenuated by the high rates of dementia at more advanced ages, and concluded that the effect of the ε4 allele might be dependent on the age of the study sample.[35]

Sekijima and colleagues examined the prevalence of DAD in 106 Japanese adults with DS aged 30 years and older.[107] They found that the frequency of the ε4 allele was approximately four times higher in demented adults with DS (18.8%) than in non-demented adults with DS (4.5%). Among those with dementia who were less than 50 years of age, the frequency of the ε4 allele was 28.6%, consistent both with a role for the ε4 allele in accelerating the onset of DAD in DS and with an age-dependent effect for the ε4 allele.

The ε4 allele has also been shown to influence the rate of cognitive decline in non-demented individuals with DS.[113,114] Alexander and colleagues compared older adults (aged 41–61 years) with young adults (22–38 years) with DS on a battery of neuropsychological tests.[113] Age-adjusted language ability – an early indicator of cognitive decline that might be associated with incipient dementia – was poorer in individuals with an ε4 allele than in those with an ε2 allele. This finding suggests that the effects of the ε4 allele may be apparent long before signs of frank dementia appear.[113] Similarly, a longitudinal analysis of cognitive performance showed a faster rate of decline in intellectual ability in adults with DS who carried at least one ε4 allele.[114]

Several meta-analyses have confirmed the effect of ApoE genotype on age at onset or risk for DAD in adults with DS.[99,101,103,105] Prasher, Lambert and colleagues failed to find a significant effect of the ε4 allele, but did find a protective effect on risk of dementia for the ε2 allele.[101,103] However, their samples included a relatively small number of individuals old enough to be at risk for dementia. Subsequent meta-analyses have included both larger and older samples in the analysis. Deb and colleagues showed that the frequency of the ε4 allele was significantly higher in demented adults with DS compared with non-demented adults (odds ratio for an ε4 allele in demented *vs.* non-demented individuals = 2.02), but there was no significant reduction in the frequency of the ε2 allele.[99] Rubinsztein and colleagues found both an increased frequency of the ε4 allele (odds ratio = 2.7) and a decreased frequency of the ε2 allele (odds ratio = 0.37) in demented compared with non-demented adults with DS.[105] Overall, the odds ratios for the age-adjusted risk of DAD range from 2 to 5 in individuals with an ε4 allele compared with those without an ε4 allele, and from 0 to 0.4 in those with an ε2 allele compared with those without an ε2 allele. These findings are consistent with reduced Aβ deposition[25] and less plaque formation[115,116] in individuals with an ε2 allele, and with acceleration of Aβ pathology in those with an ε4 allele.[24,25,117]

Telomere length and accelerated ageing

Individuals with DS have a decreased life expectancy and, as noted above, middle-aged individuals with DS show many age-related changes in health and functional status that suggest premature or accelerated ageing.[26,118] These changes include early menopause in women with DS,[119–121] early onset of senile cataracts and other sensory impairment,[122,123] hypothyroidism,[124] old-age-associated decrease in functional ability[41,125] and increased risk for DAD.[30,31,33,36,84,118,126]

Telomere length and telomerase activity may serve as important biological markers of rate of ageing in DS, and may be related to risk for dementia and other age-related disease, but have not been widely investigated. Chromosome ends or telomeres are specialised structures that consist of highly conserved series of the nucleotides thymine, adenine and guanine (TTAGGG repeats). When cells divide, telomeres are not fully replicated, and with each cell division they shorten over time, except as lengthened by telomerase.[127] Reduction in telomere length is a factor in cellular ageing related to increasing senescence, programmed cell death (apoptosis) or neoplastic transformation.[128,129] The association between telomere shortening and senescence is well established in laboratory settings, and there is increasing evidence that telomere shortening may be related to lifespan as well as to cellular ageing.[130–132] Cawthon and colleagues assessed the association between telomere length and mortality in 143 unrelated individuals.[133] They found shorter telomeres in blood DNA in individuals with poorer survival due to heart disease and infection, which suggests that telomere length may also be related to health status.[133]

Telomere length varies among individuals of the same age.[134] These individual differences may be genetically determined and influence longevity. Slagboom and colleagues[134] reported heritability estimates for telomere length of 0.78 among groups of twins ranging from 2 to 95 years in age, supporting a genetic basis for individual differences in telomere length.

Telomere length may also influence risk for AD, supporting the hypothesis that AD is related to advanced 'biological' age. A recent small study found shortening of telomeres in T-cells from 15 patients with DAD, with apparently greater shortening in individuals with lower mental status scores.[135] Vaziri and colleagues examined the rate of telomere loss in peripheral blood lymphocytes of 140 individuals ranging from 0 to 107 years in age, including 21 individuals with DS (age range 0–45 years).[136] They found that individuals with DS showed a significantly higher rate of telomere loss with age, which suggests that a reduction in telomere length may be a biomarker of accelerated ageing in individuals with DS.[136] Jenkins and colleagues found increased telomerase activity and decreased telomere length in demented compared with non-demented adults with DS (age-

and gender-matched controls).[137] These preliminary findings suggest that individual differences in telomere length or telomerase activity may be important predictors of both dementia and mortality risk.

Conclusion

Accelerated ageing and increased risk for DAD are characteristic of individuals with DS, and it is important to understand the factors that contribute to these risks. Despite the nearly universal occurrence of AD pathology by middle age, there is wide variation in age at onset of dementia, and not all adults with DS are affected. An understanding of the factors that modify age at onset of dementia can lead to the identification of critical pathogenic pathways and the development of biomarkers of risk, and can provide the basis for targeted therapeutic intervention or prevention.

Most investigators would agree that risk of DAD is raised by triplication and overexpression of the gene for APP, leading to increased formation and deposition of Aβ. Other genes that are also overexpressed by triplication of chromosome 21, such as BACE-2, SOD1 and S-100β, have received less attention but may also contribute to increased risk. Findings from studies of BACE-2 and S-100β protein appear promising, but most studies have used autopsy material and more research is needed on epidemiological samples to determine whether these findings have strong clinical significance. Most research on genetic susceptibility factors for AD in DS has focused on the role of the ApoE genotype, and there is an emerging consensus that the presence of the ApoE ϵ4 allele is associated with earlier onset and increased risk of dementia. Fewer studies have examined variants in genes such as APP or presenilins that have effects on the accumulation of cerebral Aβ.

The relationship between accelerated ageing and risk of dementia is a relatively neglected area in research on AD in adults with DS. Preliminary studies of telomere length suggest that factors which influence the rate of ageing may also influence age at onset of DAD.[136,137] For example, plasma high-density lipoprotein (HDL) levels correlate with cognitive function in centenarians.[138] Anthropometric and physiological measures (e.g. body mass index,[139,140] plasma lipids[141,142]), functional measures (e.g. lower extremity mobility[143]), health behaviours (e.g. smoking, alcohol consumption[140,144]) and intellectual functions (e.g. memory, processing speed[145-148]) each appear to have a substantial genetic influence, and have been associated with both lifespan and risk for dementia, but have not been investigated in adults with DS.

In part, the investigation of genetic and non-genetic risk factors for DAD in DS has been limited by methodological problems related to diagnosis, staging of dementia and sample characteristics (e.g. samples that are too small or too young). Reliable and valid cognitive assessment batteries and diagnostic criteria are required in order to detect dementia in the early stages and to improve studies of risk factors. At present, most diagnoses of DAD in adults with DS are made clinically and after considerable progression has already occurred, without systematic cognitive or functional testing over time. Staging of dementia will be important in the investigation of biomarkers (e.g. Aβ1–42), which can be expected to fluctuate with disease progression.

Finally, little work has been done on the interaction of susceptibility genes with risk factors or with other genes for dementia in adults with DS, and these may modulate disease phenotype as well as risk.[8] Both gene–gene interactions and interactions with non-genetic risk factors can be expected, but larger samples will be required in order to detect interactions, and a broader range of genetic, host and environmental risk factors will need to be examined.

Acknowledgements

Preparation of this paper was supported by funds provided by the New York State through its Office of Mental Retardation and Developmental Disabilities, and by grants AG014673 and HD35897 from the National Institutes of Health, and RG3–96–077 from the Alzheimer's Association.

References

1 Iwatsubo T, Odaka A, Suzuki N *et al.* (1994) Visualization of A β 42(43) and A β 40 in senile plaques with end-specific A β monoclonals: evidence that an initially deposited species is A β 42(43). *Neuron.* **13:** 45–53.

2 Younkin SG (1998) The role of A β 42 in Alzheimer's disease. *J Physiol Paris.* **92:** 289–92.

3 Cummings B and Cotman C (1995) Image analysis of β-amyloid load in Alzheimer's disease and relation to dementia severity. *Lancet.* **346:** 1524–8.

4 Jensen M, Schroder J, Blomberg M *et al.* (1999) Cerebrospinal fluid A β42 is increased early in sporadic Alzheimer's disease and declines with disease progression. *Ann Neurol.* **45:** 504–11.

5 Kanai M, Matsubara E, Isoe K *et al.* (1998) Longitudinal study of cerebrospinal fluid levels of tau, A β1–40 and A β1–42(43) in Alzheimer's disease: a study in Japan. *Ann Neurol.* **44:** 17–26.

6 Mayeux R, Honig LS, Tang MX *et al.* (2003) Plasma Aβ40 and Aβ42 and Alzheimer's disease: relation to age, mortality and risk. *Neurology.* **61:** 1185–90.

7 Mayeux R, Tang MX, Jacobs DM *et al.* (1999) Plasma amyloid β-peptide 1–42 and incipient Alzheimer's disease. *Ann Neurol.* **46:** 412–16.

8 Kennedy JL, Farrer LA, Andreasen NC *et al.* (2003) The genetics of adult-onset neuropsychiatric disease: complexities and conundra? *Science.* **302:** 822–6.

9 Goate A, Chartier-Harlin MC, Mullan M *et al.* (1991) Segregation of a missense mutation in the amyloid precursor protein gene with familial Alzheimer's disease. *Nature.* **349:** 704–6.

10 Levy-Lahad E, Wijsman EM, Nemens E *et al.* (1995). A familial Alzheimer's disease locus on chromosome 1. *Science.* **269:** 970–3.

11 Rogaev EI, Sherrington R, Rogaeva EA *et al.* (1995) Familial Alzheimer's disease in kindreds with missense mutations in a gene on chromosome 1 related to the Alzheimer's disease type 3 gene. *Nature.* **376:** 775–8.

12 Sherrington R, Rogaev EI, Liang Y *et al.* (1995) Cloning of a gene bearing missense mutations in early-onset familial Alzheimer's disease. *Nature.* **375:** 754–60.

13 Kamboh MI (2004) Molecular genetics of late-onset Alzheimer's disease. *Ann Hum Genet.* **68:** 381–404.

14 Kosaka T, Imagawa M, Seki K *et al.* (1997) The βAPP717 Alzheimer mutation increases the percentage of plasma amyloid-β protein ending at A β42(43). *Neurology.* **48:** 741–5.

15 Mann D, Iwatsubo T, Cairns J *et al.* (1996) Amyloid β protein (Aβ) deposition in chromosome-14-linked Alzheimer's disease: predominance of Aβ42(43). *Ann Neurol.* **40:** 149–56.

16 Scheuner D, Eckman C, Jensen M *et al.* (1996) Secreted amyloid beta-protein similar to that in the senile plaques of Alzheimer's disease is increased *in vivo* by the presenilin 1 and 2 and APP mutations linked to familial Alzheimer's disease. *Nat Med.* **2**: 864–70.

17 Citron M, Westaway D, Xia W *et al.* (1997) Mutant presenilins of Alzheimer's disease increase production of 42-residue amyloid beta-protein in both transfected cells and transgenic mice. *Nat Med.* **3**: 67–72.

18 Corbo RM and Scacchi R (1999) Apolipoprotein E (ApoE) allele distribution in the world. Is ApoEε4 a 'thrifty' allele? *Ann Hum Genet.* **63**: 301–10.

19 Corder EH, Saunders AM, Strittmatter WJ *et al.* (1993) Gene dose of apolipoprotein E type 4 allele and the risk of Alzheimer's disease in late-onset families. *Science.* **261**: 921–3.

20 Mayeux R, Stern Y, Ottman R *et al.* (1993) The apolipoprotein epsilon 4 allele in patients with Alzheimer's disease. *Ann Neurol.* **34**: 752–4.

21 Saunders AM, Hulette O, Welsh-Bohmer KA *et al.* (1996) Specificity, sensitivity and predictive value of apolipoprotein-E genotyping for sporadic Alzheimer's disease. *Lancet.* **348**: 90–3.

22 Strittmatter W, Saunders A, Schmechel D *et al.* (1993) Apolipoprotiein E: high-avidity binding to beta-amyloid and increased frequency of type 4-allele in late-onset familial Alzheimer disease. *Proc Natl Acad Sci USA.* **90**: 1977–81.

23 Van Duijn CM, De Knijff P, Cruts M *et al.* (1994). Apolipoprotein E4 allele in a population-based study of early-onset Alzheimer's disease. *Nat Genet.* **7**: 74–8.

24 Hyman BT, West HL, Rebeck GW *et al.* (1995) Quantitative analysis of senile plaques in Alzheimer disease: observation of log-normal size distribution and molecular epidemiology of differences associated with apolipoprotein E genotype and trisomy 21 (Down syndrome). *Proc Natl Acad Sci USA.* **92**: 3586–90.

25 Polvikoski T, Sulkhava R, Haltia M *et al.* (1995) Apolipoprotein E, dementia, and cortical deposition of beta-amyloid protein. *NEJM.* **333**: 1242–7.

26 Martin GM (1979) Genetic and evolutionary aspects of aging. *Fed Proc.* **38**: 1962–7.

27 Malamud N (1972) Neuropathology of organic brain syndromes associated with aging. In: CM Gaitz (ed.) *Ageing and the Brain: advances in behavioural biology.* Plenum, New York.

28 Wisniewski KE, Wisniewski HM and Wen GY (1985) Occurrence of neuropathological changes and dementia of Alzheimer's disease in Down's syndrome. *Ann Neurol.* **17**: 278–82.

29 Rumble B, Retallack R, Hilbich C *et al.* (1989) Amyloid A4 protein and its precursor in Down's syndrome and Alzheimer's disease. *NEJM.* **320**: 1446–52.

30 Schupf N (2002) Genetic and host factors for dementia in Down's syndrome. *Br J Psychiatry.* **180**: 405–10.

31 Zigman W, Schupf N, Haveman M *et al.* (1997) The epidemiology of Alzheimer disease in intellectual disability: results and recommendations from an international conference. *J Intellect Disabil Res.* **41**: 76–80.

32 Devenny DA, Krinsky-McHale SJ, Sersen G *et al.* (2000) Sequence of cognitive decline in dementia in adults with Down's syndrome. *J Intellect Disabil Res.* **44**: 654–65.

33 Holland AJ, Hon J, Huppert FA *et al.* (1998) Population-based study of the prevalence and presentation of dementia in adults with Down's syndrome. *Br J Psychiatry.* **172**: 493–8.

34 Hon J, Huppert FA, Holland AJ *et al.* (1999) Neuropsychological assessment of older adults with Down's syndrome: an epidemiological study using the Cambridge Cognitive Examination (CAMCOG). *Br J Clin Psychol.* **38**: 155–65.

35 Lai F, Kammann E, Rebeck GW *et al.* (1999) ApoE genotype and gender effects on Alzheimer disease in 100 adults with Down syndrome. *Neurology.* **53**: 331–6.

36 Lai F and Williams RS (1989) A prospective study of Alzheimer disease in Down syndrome. *Arch Neurol.* **46**: 849–53.

37 Prasher VP, Chung MC and Haque MS (1998) Longitudinal changes in adaptive behavior in adults with Down syndrome: interim findings from a longitudinal study. *Am J Ment Retard.* **103**: 40–6.

38 Prasher VP and Krishnan VH (1993) Mental disorders and adaptive behaviour in people with Down's syndrome. *Br J Psychiatry.* **162**: 848–50.

39 Thase ME, Tigner R, Smeltzer DJ *et al.* (1984) Age-related neuropsychological deficits in Down's syndrome. *Biol Psychiatry.* **19**: 571–85.

40 Visser FE, Aldenkamp AP, Van Huffelen AC *et al.* (1997) Prospective study of the prevalence of Alzheimer-type dementia in institutionalized individuals with Down syndrome. *Am J Ment Retard.* **101**: 400–12.

41 Zigman WB, Schupf N, Lubin RA *et al.* (1987) Premature regression of adults with Down syndrome. *Am J Ment Defic.* **92**: 161–8.

42 Wisniewski HM, Wegiel J and Popovitch E (1994) Age-associated development of diffuse and thioflavin-S-positive plaques in Down syndrome. *Dev Brain Dysfunction.* **7**: 330–9.

43 Borchelt DR, Thinakaran G, Eckman CB *et al.* (1996) Familial Alzheimer's disease-linked presenilin 1 variants elevate Aβ1–42/1–40 ratio *in vitro* and *in vivo*. *Neuron.* **17**: 1005–13.

44 Younkin SG (1997) The AAP and PS1/2 mutations linked to early-onset familial Alzheimer's disease increase the extracellular concentration and A β 1–42 (43). *Rinsho Shinkeigaku.* **37**: 1099.

45 Ertekin-Taner N, Graff-Radford N, Younkin LH *et al.* (2001) Heritability of plasma amyloid beta in typical late-onset Alzheimer's disease pedigrees. *Genet Epidemiol.* **21**: 19–30.

46 Ertekin-Taner N, Graff-Radford N, Younkin LH *et al.* (2000) Linkage of plasma Aβ42 to a quantitative locus on chromosome 10 in late-onset Alzheimer's disease pedigrees. *Science.* **290**: 2303–5.

47 Kehoe P, Wavrant-De Vrieze F, Crook R *et al.* (1999) A full genome scan for late-onset Alzheimer's disease. *Hum Mol Genet.* **8**: 237–45.

48 Myers A, Holmans P, Marshall H *et al.* (2000) Susceptibility locus for Alzheimer's disease on chromosome 10. *Science.* **290**: 2304–5.

49 Iwatsubo T, Mann DM, Odaka A *et al.* (1995) Amyloid beta protein (Aβ) deposition: A β 42(43) precedes A β 40 in Down syndrome. *Ann Neurol.* **37**: 294–9.

50 Teller JK, Russo C, DeBusk LM *et al.* (1996) Presence of soluble amyloid beta-peptide precedes amyloid plaque formation in Down's syndrome. *Nat Med.* **2**: 93–5.

51 Prasher VP, Farrer MJ, Kessling AM *et al.* (1998) Molecular mapping of Alzheimer-type dementia in Down's syndrome. *Ann Neurol.* **43**: 380–3.

52 Cavani S, Tamaoka A, Moretti A *et al.* (2000) Plasma levels of amyloid β 40 and 42 are independent from ApoE genotype and mental retardation in Down syndrome. *Am J Med Genet.* **95**: 224–8.

53 Mehta PD, Dalton AJ, Mehta SP *et al.* (1998) Increased plasma amyloid β protein 1–42 levels in Down syndrome. *Neurosci Lett.* **241**: 13–16.

54 Schupf N, Patel B, Silverman W *et al.* (2001) Elevated plasma amyloid beta-peptide 1–42 and onset of dementia in adults with Down syndrome. *Neurosci Lett.* **301**: 199–203.

55 Tokuda T, Fukushima T, Ikeda S *et al.* (1997) Plasma levels of amyloid beta proteins Aβ1–40 and Aβ1–42(43) are elevated in Down's syndrome. *Ann Neurol.* **41**: 271–3.

56 Mehta PD, Mehta SP, Fedor B *et al.* (2003) Plasma amyloid beta protein 1–42 levels are increased in old Down syndrome but not in young Down syndrome. *Neurosci Lett.* **342**: 155–8.

57 Ma J, Yee A, Brewer HB Jr *et al.* (1994) Amyloid-associated proteins alpha-1-antichymotrypsin and apolipoprotein E promote assembly of Alzheimer beta-protein into filaments. *Nature.* **372**: 92–4.

58 McNamara MJ, Gomez-Isla T and Hyman BT (1998) Apolipoprotein E genotype and deposits of Aβ40 and Aβ42 in Alzheimer disease. *Arch Neurol.* **55**: 1001–4.

59 Tapiola T, Soininen H and Pirttila T (2001) CSF tau and Aβ42 levels in patients with Down's syndrome. *Neurology.* **56**: 979–80.

60 Tapiola T, Pirttila T, Mehta PD *et al.* (2000) Relationship between apoE genotype and CSF beta-amyloid (1–42) and tau in patients with probable and definite Alzheimer's disease. *Neurobiol Aging.* **21**: 735–40.

61 Barbiero L, Benussi L, Ghidoni R *et al.* (2003) BACE-2 is overexpressed in Down's syndrome. *Exp Neurol.* **182**: 335–45.

62 Motonaga K, Itoh M, Becker LE *et al.* (2002) Elevated expression of beta-site amyloid precursor protein cleaving enzyme 2 in brains of patients with Down syndrome. *Neurosci Lett.* **326**: 64–6.

63 Head E and Lott IT (2004) Down syndrome and beta-amyloid deposition. *Curr Opin Neurol.* **17**: 95–100.

64 Castets F, Griffin WS, Marks A *et al.* (1997) Transcriptional regulation of the human S100 beta gene. *Brain Res Mol Brain Res.* **46**: 208–16.

65 Shapiro LA, Marks A and Whitaker-Azmitia PM (2004) Increased clusterin expression in old but not young adult S100B transgenic mice: evidence of neuropathological aging in a model of Down syndrome. *Brain Res.* **1010**: 17–21.

66 Griffin WS, Sheng JG, McKenzie JE *et al.* (1998). Life-long overexpression of S100beta in Down's syndrome: implications for Alzheimer pathogenesis. *Neurobiol Aging.* **19**: 401–5.

67 Li Y, Wang J, Sheng JG *et al.* (1998) S100 beta increases levels of beta-amyloid precursor protein and its encoding mRNA in rat neuronal cultures. *J Neurochem.* **71**: 1421–8.

68 Mrak RE, Sheng JG and Griffin WS (1996) Correlation of astrocytic S100 beta expression with dystrophic neurites in amyloid plaques of Alzheimer's disease. *J Neuropathol Exp Neurol.* **55**: 273–9.

69 Sheng JG, Mrak RE, Rovnaghi CR *et al.* (1996) Human brain S100 beta and S100 beta mRNA expression increases with age: pathogenic implications for Alzheimer's disease. *Neurobiol Aging.* **17**: 359–63.

70 Sheng JG, Mrak RE and Griffin WS (1994) S100 beta protein expression in Alzheimer disease: potential role in the pathogenesis of neuritic plaques. *J Neurosci Res.* **39**: 398–404.

71 Becker L, Mito T, Takashima S *et al.* (1993) Association of phenotypic abnormalities of Down syndrome with an imbalance of genes on chromosome 21. *APMIS.* **Suppl. 40**: 57–70.

72 Mito T and Becker LE (1993) Developmental changes of S-100 protein and glial fibrillary acidic protein in the brain in Down syndrome. *Exp Neurol.* **120**: 170–6.

73 Whitaker-Azmitia PM, Wingate M, Borella A *et al.* (1997) Transgenic mice over-expressing the neurotrophic factor S-100 beta show neuronal cytoskeletal and behavioral signs of altered aging processes: implications for Alzheimer's disease and Down's syndrome. *Brain Res.* **776**: 51–60.

74 Mrak RE and Griffin WS (2004) Trisomy 21 and the brain. *J Neuropathol Exp Neurol.* **63**: 679–85.

75 De La Monte SM (1999) Molecular abnormalities of the brain in Down syndrome: relevance to Alzheimer's neurodegeneration. *J Neural Transm.* **Suppl. 57**: 1–19.

76 Shapiro LA and Whitaker-Azmitia PM (2004) Expression levels of cytoskeletal proteins indicate pathological aging of S100B transgenic mice: an immunohistochemical study of MAP-2, drebrin and GAP-43. *Brain Res.* **1019**: 39–46.

77 Winocur G, Roder J and Lobaugh N (2001) Learning and memory in S100-beta transgenic mice: an analysis of impaired and preserved function. *Neurobiol Learn Mem.* **75**: 230–43.

78 Royston MC, McKenzie JE, Gentleman SM *et al.* (1999) Overexpression of s100beta in Down's syndrome: correlation with patient age and with beta-amyloid deposition. *Neuropathol Appl Neurobiol.* **25**: 387–93.

79 Athan ES, Lee JH, Arriaga A *et al.* (2002) Polymorphisms in the promoter of the human APP gene: functional evaluation and allele frequencies in Alzheimer disease. *Arch Neurol.* **59**: 1793–9.

80 Margallo-Lana M, Morris CM, Gibson AM *et al.* (2004) Influence of the amyloid precursor protein locus on dementia in Down syndrome. *Neurology.* **62**: 1996–8.

81 Lucarelli P, Piciullo A, Palmarino M *et al.* (2004) Association between presenilin-1 -48T/C polymorphism and Down's syndrome. *Neurosci Lett.* **367**: 88–91.

82 Tyrrell J, Cosgrave M, McPherson J *et al.* (1999) Presenilin 1 and alpha-1-anti-chymotrypsin polymorphisms in Down syndrome: no effect on the presence of dementia. *Am J Med Genet.* **88**: 616–20.

83 Pollwein P, Masters CL and Beyreuther K (1992) The expression of the amyloid precursor protein (APP) is regulated by two GC-elements in the promoter. *Nucleic Acids Res.* **20**: 63–8.

84 Holland AJ, Hon J, Huppert FA *et al.* (2000) Incidence and course of dementia in people with Down's syndrome: findings from a population-based study. *J Intellect Disabil Res.* **44**: 138–46.

85 Zigman WB, Schupf N, Sersen E *et al.* (1996) Prevalence of dementia in adults with and without Down syndrome. *Am J Ment Retard.* **100**: 403–12.

86 Mahley RW (1988) Apolipoprotein E: cholesterol transport protein with expanding role in cell biology. *Science.* **240**: 622–30.

87 Davignon J, Gregg RE and Sing CF (1988). Apolipoprotein E polymorphism and atherosclerosis. *Arteriosclerosis.* **8**: 1–21.

88 Schupf N, Kapell D, Lee JH *et al.* (1996) Onset of dementia is associated with apolipoprotein E epsilon 4 in Down's syndrome. *Ann Neurol.* **40**: 799–801.

89 Schachter F, Faure-Delanef L, Guenot F *et al.* (1994) Genetic associations with human longevity at the APOE and ACE loci. *Nat Genet.* **6**: 29–32.

90 Hirose N, Homma S, Arai Y *et al.* (1997) Tokyo Centenarian Study. 4. Apolipoprotein E phenotype in Japanese centenarians living in the Tokyo Metropolitan area. *Nippon Ronen Igakkai Zasshi.* **34**: 267–72.

91 Louhija J, Miettinen HE, Kontula K *et al.* (1994) Aging and genetic variation of plasma apolipoproteins. Relative loss of the apolipoprotein E4 phenotype in centenarians. *Arterioscler Thromb Vasc Biol.* **14**: 1084–9.

92 Lee JH, Tang MX, Schupf N *et al.* (2001) Mortality and apolipoprotein E in Hispanic, African-American and Caucasian elders. *Am J Med Genet.* **103**: 121–7.

93 Bader G, Zuliani G, Kostner GM *et al.* (1998) Apolipoprotein E polymorphism is not associated with longevity or disability in a sample of Italian octo- and nonagenarians. *Gerontology.* **44**: 293–9.

94 Galinsky D, Tysoe C, Brayne CE *et al.* (1997) Analysis of the apo E/apo C-I, angiotensin-converting enzyme and methylenetetrahydrofolate reductase genes as candidates affecting human longevity. *Atherosclerosis.* **129**: 177–83.

95 Jian-Gang Z, Yong-Xing M, Chuan-Fu W *et al.* (1998) Apolipoprotein E and longevity among Han Chinese population. *Mech Ageing Dev.* **104**: 159–67.

96 Corder EH, Saunders AM, Risch NJ *et al.* (1994) Protective effect of apolipoprotein E type 2 allele for late-onset Alzheimer disease. *Nat Genet.* **7**: 180–4.

97 Roses AD (1994) Apolipoprotein E affects the rate of Alzheimer disease expression: beta-amyloid burden is a secondary consequence dependent on ApoE genotype and duration of disease. *J Neuropathol Exp Neurol.* **53**: 429–37.

98 Cosgrave M, Tyrrell J, Dreja H *et al.* (1996) Lower frequency of apolipoprotein E4 allele in an 'elderly' Down's syndrome population. *Biol Psychiatry.* **40**: 811–13.

 99 Deb S, Braganza J, Norton N *et al.* (2000) ApoE epsilon 4 influences the manifestation of Alzheimer's disease in adults with Down's syndrome. *Br J Psychiatry.* **176:** 468–72.

100 Hardy J, Crook R, Perry R *et al.* (1994) ApoE genotype and Down's syndrome [letter]. *Lancet.* **343:** 979–80.

101 Lambert JC, Perez-Tur J, Dupire MJ *et al.* (1996) Analysis of the ApoE alleles: impact in Down's syndrome. *Neurosci Lett.* **220:** 57–60.

102 Martins RN, Clarnette R, Fisher C *et al.* (1995) ApoE genotypes in Australia: roles in early- and late-onset Alzheimer's disease and Down's syndrome. *Neuroreport.* **6:** 1513–16.

103 Prasher VP, Chowdhury TA, Rowe BR *et al.* (1997) ApoE genotype and Alzheimer's disease in adults with Down syndrome: meta-analysis. *Am J Ment Retard.* **102:** 103–10.

104 Royston MC, Mann D, Pickering-Brown S *et al.* (1994) Apolipoprotein E epsilon 2 allele promotes longevity and protects patients with Down's syndrome from dementia. *Neuroreport.* **5:** 2583–5.

105 Rubinsztein DC, Hon J, Stevens F *et al.* (1999) Apo E genotypes and risk of dementia in Down syndrome. *Am J Med Genet.* **88:** 344–7.

106 Schupf N, Kapell D, Nightingale B *et al.* (1998) Earlier onset of Alzheimer's disease in men with Down syndrome. *Neurology.* **50:** 991–5.

107 Sekijima Y, Ikeda S, Tokuda T *et al.* (1998) Prevalence of dementia of Alzheimer type and apolipoprotein E phenotypes in aged patients with Down's syndrome. *Eur Neurol.* **39:** 234–7.

108 Tyrrell J, Cosgrave M, Hawi Z *et al.* (1998) A protective effect of apolipoprotein E ϵ2 allele on dementia in Down's syndrome. *Biol Psychiatry.* **43:** 397–400.

109 Van Gool WA, Evenhuis HM and Van Duijn CM (1995) A case–control study of apolipoprotein E genotypes in Alzheimer's disease associated with Down's syndrome. Dutch Study Group on Down's Syndrome and Ageing. *Ann Neurol.* **38:** 225–30.

110 Holder JL, Habbak RA, Pearlson GD *et al.* (1996) Reduced survival of apolipoprotein E4 homozygotes in Down's syndrome? *Neuroreport.* **7:** 2455–6.

111 Edland SD, Wijsman EM, Schoder-Ehri GL *et al.* (1997) Little evidence of reduced survival to adulthood of apoE epsilon4 homozygotes in Down's syndrome. *Neuroreport.* **8:** 3463–5.

112 Saunders AM, Strittmatter WJ, Schmechel D *et al.* (1993) Association of apolipoprotein E allele epsilon 4 with late-onset familial and sporadic Alzheimer's disease. *Neurology.* **43:** 1467–72.

113 Alexander GE, Saunders AM, Szczepanik J *et al.* (1997) Relation of age and apolipoprotein E to cognitive function in Down syndrome adults. *Neuroreport.* **8:** 1835–40.

114 Del Bo R, Comi GP, Bresolin N *et al.* (1997) The apolipoprotein E epsilon4 allele causes a faster decline of cognitive performances in Down's syndrome subjects. *J Neurol Sci.* **145:** 87–91.

115 Benjamin R, Leake A, McArthur FK *et al.* (1994) Protective effect of apoE epsilon 2 in Alzheimer's disease. *Lancet.* **344:** 473.

116 Lippa CF, Smith TW, Saunders AM *et al.* (1997) Apolipoprotein E-epsilon 2 and Alzheimer's disease: genotype influences pathologic phenotype. *Neurology.* **48:** 515–19.

117 Hyman BT (1992) Down syndrome and Alzheimer disease. *Prog Clin Biol Res.* **379:** 123–42.

118 Oliver C and Holland AJ (1986) Down's syndrome and Alzheimer's disease: a review. *Psychol Med.* **16:** 307–22.

119 Carr J and Hollins S (1995) Menopause in women with learning disabilities. *J Intellect Disabil Res.* **39:** 137–9.

120 Schupf N, Zigman W, Kapell D *et al.* (1997) Early menopause in women with Down's syndrome. *J Intellect Disabil Res.* **41:** 264–7.

121 Seltzer GB, Schupf N and Wu HS (2001) A prospective study of menopause in women with Down's syndrome. *J Intellect Disabil Res.* **45:** 1–7.

122 Evenhuis HM, Theunissen M, Denkers I et al. (2001) Prevalence of visual and hearing impairment in a Dutch institutionalized population with intellectual disability. *J Intellect Disabil Res.* **45:** 457–64.

123 Van Schrojenstein Lantman-de Valk HM, Haveman MJ, Maaskant MA et al. (1994) The need for assessment of sensory functioning in ageing people with mental handicap. *J Intellect Disabil Res.* **38:** 289–98.

124 Kapell D, Nightingale B, Rodriguez A et al. (1998) Prevalence of chronic medical conditions in adults with mental retardation: comparison with the general population. *Ment Retard.* **36:** 269–79.

125 Prasher VP and Chung MC (1996) Causes of age-related decline in adaptive behavior of adults with Down syndrome: differential diagnoses of dementia. *Am J Ment Retard.* **101:** 175–83.

126 Oliver C, Crayton L, Holland A et al. (1998) A four-year prospective study of age-related cognitive change in adults with Down's syndrome. *Psychol Med.* **28:** 1365–77.

127 Chan SR and Blackburn EH (2004) Telomeres and telomerase. *Philos Trans R Soc Lond B Biol Sci.* **359:** 109–21.

128 Rubin H (1997) Cell aging *in vivo* and *in vitro*. *Mech Ageing Dev.* **98:** 1–35.

129 Shay JW and Wright WE (2001) *Ageing and Cancer: the telomere and telomerase connection.* Novartis Foundation Symposium, London.

130 Ahmed A and Tollefsbol T (2001) Telomeres and telomerase: basic science implications for aging. *J Am Geriatr Soc.* **49:** 1105–9.

131 Frenck RW Jr, Blackburn EH and Shannon KM (1998) The rate of telomere sequence loss in human leukocytes varies with age. *Proc Natl Acad Sci USA.* **95:** 5607–10.

132 Londono-Vallejo JA, DerSarkissian H, Cazes L et al. (2001) Differences in telomere length between homologous chromosomes in humans. *Nucleic Acids Res.* **29:** 3164–71.

133 Cawthon RM, Smith KR, O'Brien E et al. (2003) Association between telomere length in blood and mortality in people aged 60 years or older. *Lancet.* **361:** 393–5.

134 Slagboom PE, Droog S and Boomsma DI (1994) Genetic determination of telomere size in humans: a twin study of three age groups. *Am J Hum Genet.* **55:** 876–82.

135 Panossian LA, Porter VR, Valenzuela HF et al. (2003) Telomere shortening in T-cells correlates with Alzheimer's disease status. *Neurobiol Aging.* **24:** 77–84.

136 Vaziri H, Schachter F, Uchida I et al. (1993) Loss of telomeric DNA during aging of normal and trisomy 21 human lymphocytes. *Am J Hum Genet.* **52:** 661–7.

137 Jenkins E, Velinov M, Li S-Y et al. (2002) Increased telomerase activity in older individuals with Down syndrome and dementia. *Am J Hum Genet.* **71:** 351A.

138 Atzmon G, Gabriely I, Greiner W et al. (2002) Plasma HDL levels highly correlate with cognitive function in exceptional longevity. *J Gerontol A Biol Sci Med Sci.* **57:** M712–15.

139 Austin MA, Friedlander Y, Newman B et al. (1997) Genetic influences on changes in body mass index: a longitudinal analysis of women twins. *Obes Res.* **5:** 326–31.

140 Herskind AM, McGue M, Iachine IA et al. (1996) Untangling genetic influences on smoking, body mass index and longevity: a multivariate study of 2464 Danish twins followed for 28 years. *Hum Genet.* **98:** 467–75.

141 Heller DA, Pedersen NL, deFaire U et al. (1994) Genetic and environmental correlations among serum lipids and apolipoproteins in elderly twins reared together and apart. *Am J Hum Genet.* **55:** 1255–67.

142 Snieder H, Van Doornen LJ and Boomsma DI (1997) The age dependency of gene expression for plasma lipids, lipoproteins and apolipoproteins. *Am J Hum Genet.* **60:** 638–50.

143 Carmelli D, DeCarli C, Swan GE et al. (2000) The joint effect of apolipoprotein E epsilon 4 and MRI findings on lower-extremity function and decline in cognitive function. *J Gerontol A Biol Sci Med Sci.* **55:** M103–9.

144 Almasy L and Borecki IB (1999) Exploring genetic analysis of complex traits through the paradigm of alcohol dependence: summary of GAW11 contribution. *Genet Epidemiol.* **17:** S1–24.

145 Finkel D, Pedersen N and McGue M (1995) Genetic influences on memory performance in adulthood: comparison of Minnesota and Swedish twin data. *Psychol Aging.* **10:** 437–46.

146 Finkel D, Pedersen NL, McGue M *et al.* (1995) Heritability of cognitive abilities in adult twins: comparison of Minnesota and Swedish data. *Behav Genet.* **25:** 421–31.

147 Reed T, Carmelli D, Swan GE *et al.* (1994) Lower cognitive performance in normal older adult male twins carrying the apolipoprotein E epsilon 4 allele. *Arch Neurol.* **51:** 1189–92.

148 Swan GE, Reed T, Jack LM *et al.* (1999) Differential genetic influence for components of memory in aging adult twins. *Arch Neurol.* **56:** 1127–32.

Chapter 4

Amyloid beta and tau proteins in Alzheimer's disease and Down syndrome

Pankaj D Mehta

Introduction

Alzheimer's disease (AD) is one of the commonest dementing illnesses, affecting about four million people in the USA. It is characterised clinically not only by an impairment in cognition but also by a decline in global function, a deterioration in the ability to perform activities of daily living, and the appearance of behavioural disturbances.[1,2] The average course of dementia in Alzheimer's disease (DAD) is approximately a decade, but the rate of progression is variable. Approximately 8–10% of all individuals over 65 years of age have DAD, and the prevalence of the disease doubles every five years after the age of 65 years.

The primary risk factors for DAD are age and family history. While the majority of DAD cases are sporadic, approximately 5% of cases are familial with autosomal-dominant inheritance. Although the aetiology of AD is not known, genetic factors play a major role. Early-onset DAD is caused by defects in one of three genes – presenilin 1 (PS1) on chromosome 14, presenilin 2 (PS2) on chromosome 1 and amyloid precursor protein (APP) on chromosome 21.[3]

Apolipoprotein E (ApoE) is a 34-kDa polymorphic protein that is involved in the transport and redistribution of lipids among various tissues. ApoE occurs as three major isoforms (E2, E3 and E4) and is encoded by three alleles (ϵ2, ϵ3 and ϵ4) at the ApoE locus on chromosome 19. The ApoE ϵ4 allele is a significant risk factor for the development of sporadic and familial late-onset DAD.[4,5]

Neurofibrillary tangles (NFT) and amyloid-bearing neuritic plaques in the limbic and cerebral cortices are the characteristic neuropathological lesions in AD brains.[6,7] A large number of neurons in AD brain that bear NFT are composed of paired helical filaments (PHF). The major component of PHF is the microtubule-associated protein tau in an abnormally phosphorylated form. The major component of neuritic plaques is the amyloid β-peptide (Aβ), a small 42-residue protein formed by proteolytic processing of a larger membrane-bound glycoprotein, the APP.[6] Secreted soluble Aβ is a product of normal cell metabolism and is found in various body fluids, including plasma and cerebrospinal fluid (CSF).[8–10] Recent studies have shown that in AD brain, Aβ ending at residue 42 (Aβ42) is deposited first and is the predominant form in senile plaques, whereas Aβ ending at residue 40 (Aβ40) is deposited later in the disease and is prominent in vascular amyloid deposits.[7] Accumulating data support the central role of Aβ42 in the formation of neuritic plaques.[11] Of all the Aβ that is normally released from cells, Aβ40 accounts for approximately 90% while Aβ42 accounts for approximately 10%.

The diagnosis of DAD is generally made by clinical evaluations and exclusion of other causes of dementia. Without histopathological confirmation of the autopsy brain tissue, the diagnosis cannot be made with certainty. Studies of the histopathological correlation have shown an accuracy of more than 85%, based on the criteria of the National Institute of Neurological and Communicative Diseases and Stroke/Alzheimer's Disease and Related Disorders Association (NINCDS–ADRDA).[12] At present, there is no specific laboratory test available to support the diagnosis of probable DAD.

Recent studies have identified a state between the cognitive changes of normal ageing and DAD, known as mild cognitive impairment (MCI).[13] Although individuals with MCI experience memory loss to a greater extent than one would expect for their age, they do not meet the criteria of probable DAD.

A biological marker confirms the presence or absence of a given disease or identifies presymptomatic individuals who are at high risk of developing a disease. A marker may reflect the primary pathogenesis of the disease or secondary processes involved in the progression of the disease, or it may be an epiphenomenon. There are two major directions in which to search for diagnostic and progression markers in AD:

1 neuroimaging techniques, which provide structural or metabolic information about the brain and identify brain atrophy changes for monitoring progression of the disease
2 several CSF measurements appear to be useful as diagnostic markers.

Blood, CSF and peripheral tissues have been examined in an attempt to find a biochemical marker for the diagnosis of probable DAD in living patients. This chapter focuses on the measurement of blood or CSF tau protein and of Aβ in individuals with Down syndrome (DS) and AD.

Relationship between brain and CSF

About 70–80% of CSF is produced in the choroid plexus of the brain ventricles, and additional CSF is formed from the brain extracellular fluid (ECF).[14] Brain ECF is in direct contact with CSF via patent ependymal and pial surfaces along the ventriculo-subarachnoid space, and the molecules entering brain ECF will eventually diffuse into the CSF. Both ECF and CSF serve as an intracerebral transport mechanism to permit diffusion of substances released by neurons and glia. The protein composition of CSF is likely to reflect that of the brain intercellular spaces, and therefore the CSF examination provides a way to sample the microenvironment of the brain.

Tau protein in CSF and plasma

Tau is an endogenous microtubule-associated phosphoprotein, located mainly in axons, which regulates the polymerisation of microtubule monomers, resulting in stabilisation of the microtubules. Tau exists in six isoforms, which are derived by alternative splicing.[15] It is mainly synthesised in neurons,[16] but is also present in astrocytes[17] and oligodendrocytes,[18] and in peripheral tissues.[19]

Secreted tau protein can be detected in CSF under normal conditions.[20] CSF tau consists of variable tau protein fragments with molecular weights ranging from 14 kDa to 68 kDa.[20–25] However, the source of CSF tau is unknown. The levels are not dependent upon blood–brain barrier dysfunction.[26] It has been suggested that increased levels of CSF tau reflect the neurofibrillary pathology in brain tissue,[27] or a more general phenomenon of axonal degeneration and neuronal cell death.[28] Studies that included controls covering a wide age range have shown that CSF tau levels increase with age,[20,29–31] whereas other studies that used controls with a limited age range have shown no significant change.[23,28,32]

Since the study by Vandermeeren and colleagues[33] that first showed increased total tau levels in CSF of patients with DAD, over 40 different studies have been published. At least three different enzyme-linked immunosorbent assay (ELISA) methods have been described.[23,28,33] All of the studies have confirmed that there is an increase in total CSF tau protein concentration in patients with AD compared with controls.[20,23,28,30,32,34–41] The sensitivity ranged from 50% to 90% and the specificity ranged from 60% to 90% for discriminating DAD from controls and non-DAD dementias. The low sensitivity may be related to differences in patient populations. Significant correlations between the ApoE genotype and CSF tau levels have also been found in some studies,[32,41–43] while others have found no association between ApoE genotype and CSF tau levels.[21,34–36,44–47]

Increased levels of CSF tau are not specific for DAD, and have been found in patients with other neurological diseases and non-DAD dementias. The highest levels of CSF were reported in patients with head trauma[25] and Creutzfeldt–Jakob disease.[48,49] A transient increase in total tau levels in CSF can also be detected up to three weeks after acute stroke.[50] These findings support the hypothesis that CSF tau may be a marker of neuronal cell death and axonal degeneration.[25,28]

Many studies have shown that CSF tau levels increase early in the course of DAD[32,41,46, 51,52] and may predict the development of DAD in patients with MCI.[53] However, the relationship between CSF tau levels and progression of the disease is controversial. Some cross-sectional studies have shown a correlation between CSF tau concentration and the severity of dementia,[30,54] but most studies have found no association.[20,32,35,36,40,41,44,46,51,52,55] Longitudinal studies have also yielded controversial results. Isoe and colleagues[56] reported that CSF tau levels were increased up to the mid-stage of DAD and decreased at the late stage. In contrast, other studies found no change.[47,57,58] In conclusion, the increase in CSF tau levels in patients with DAD is well established. However, the test is not specific because of the overlap seen among patients with DAD, those with non-DAD dementias and those with other neurological diseases.

Phospho-tau

Studies have suggested that phosphorylation of tau is an early event in AD pathogenesis.[59] These data prompted the development of methods for measurement of phosphorylated tau in CSF. Promising efforts are currently under way to establish phospho-tau (p-tau) in CSF as a putative disease-specific biological marker for AD. Immunoassays have been developed that specifically detect tau at different epitopes, such as threonine 231 (p-tau$_{231}$), serine 199 (p-tau$_{199}$) and threonine 181 (p-tau$_{181}$).[60] Evidence from these studies indicates that quantification of tau phosphorylated at these specific sites may improve early detection, differential diagnosis and tracking of disease progression in DAD.

In a pilot study, CSF p-tau$_{231}$ distinguished between individuals with DAD and those with other neurological disorders, with a sensitivity of 85% and a specificity of 97%.[61] In an independent large-scale multi-centre study, p-tau$_{231}$ significantly improved the differential diagnosis between DAD and other non-DAD groups (sensitivity of 90% and specificity of 80%). In DAD *vs.* fronto-temporal dementia, p-tau$_{231}$ raised sensitivity levels compared with t-tau from 57.7% to 90.2% at a specificity level of 92.3% for both markers.[62] In the differentiation between DAD and geriatric major depression, specificity levels were raised from 68% for t-tau to 85% using p-tau$_{231}$ at a sensitivity level of 90% for both markers. The discriminative power of p-tau$_{231}$ was significantly higher than that of t-tau.[63] Itoh and colleagues reported that CSF p-tau$_{199}$ discriminates between DAD and a combined group of non-DAD subjects with a sensitivity and specificity of 85%.[64] CSF p-tau$_{181}$ was elevated in DAD compared with other dementias and healthy controls, and has been proposed as a potential marker for discriminating individuals with DAD from those suffering from dementia with Lewy bodies[31] or vascular dementia. In a six-year serial CSF longitudinal study, p-tau$_{231}$ concentrations decreased linearly with time in patients with DAD. Furthermore, the rate of change of p-tau$_{231}$ concentration was correlated with the Mini Mental State Examination (MMSE) score at baseline, with a more pronounced rate of decline with advanced cognitive impairment. This was not found for t-tau.[65] Another promising application of p-tau$_{231}$ may be its ability to predict cognitive decline and conversion from MCI to DAD. A one-year longitudinal MCI study showed progressive elevation of p-tau$_{231}$ levels in MCI subjects compared with healthy controls.[66] High CSF p-tau$_{231}$ levels were significantly correlated with subsequent cognitive decline and conversion to DAD. In addition to p-tau$_{231}$ concentration, old age and ApoE ϵ4 carrier status independently predicted cognitive decline in this sample of 77 MCI subjects. The whole model explained 27% of the variance.[62] Confirmation of assay performance at autopsy in prospective, population-based studies is warranted in order to fully establish CSF p-tau proteins as putative specific AD biomarkers for routine diagnostic use. To compare diagnostic accuracy and combined evaluation of CSF concentrations of p-tau$_{231}$, p-tau$_{181}$ and p-tau$_{199}$, a large-scale multi-centre comparative study is essential.

Several reports[19,67] have shown that tau protein is present not only within the central nervous system but also in peripheral tissues. However, most studies could not detect tau levels in plasma from patients with DAD or from controls. One study reported tau or tau-like immunoreactivity in 20% of human plasma.[68] Further characterisation is needed in order to determine whether this protein is a member of the tau family.

Aβ in CSF

The core protein of neuritic plaques is a 4-kDa peptide, Aβ, which is proteolytically derived from the larger transmembrane glycoprotein, APP.[6] Soluble forms of Aβ generated from the APP commonly end at C-terminal residue 40 (Aβ40) or 42 (Aβ42). Immunohistochemical studies have shown that Aβ42 is predominantly associated with parenchymal amyloid of both the core-containing and the diffuse type, while Aβ40 is found occasionally with core deposits but not with the diffuse amyloid form.[69] The changes in levels of total Aβ in CSF have been extensively studied in patients with DAD and in controls. The results were controversial, showing a decrease,[70] an increase[71] or no change.[36,72–74] Our studies demonstrated that CSF levels of total Aβ are lower in patients with severe congophilic angiopathy than in those with mild to moderate angiopathy.[75]

Recent studies have focused on measurements of different isoforms of Aβ in CSF, particularly Aβ42, due to its critical role in the early pathogenesis of AD. Many different home-made ELISA tests have been developed for measuring Aβ42 in CSF and plasma,[36,76–78] and there is currently one commercially available ELISA kit for measuring Aβ42 in CSF.[79] These tests employ different antibodies, which may partially explain the differences in the results. Since Motter and colleagues first showed in 1995 that Aβ42 concentrations are decreased in CSF of patients with DAD, a number of studies have confirmed this finding.[30,32,34,35,48,58,79–84] The specificity for distinguishing patients with DAD from controls has varied from 42% to 88%, and the sensitivity has varied from 72% to 100% in these studies. We found that the Aβ42 levels were lower in patients with DAD who carried the ApoE ϵ4 allele than in those without the ApoE ϵ4 allele.[41] The sensitivity of Aβ42 measurement was 83.6% for patients with DAD who carried the ApoE ϵ4 allele, whereas in patients with DAD without the ApoE ϵ4 allele it was 54.2%. Several studies have confirmed that there is a significant association between CSF Aβ42 levels and the ApoE genotype.[32,35] There is strong evidence that Aβ deposits are more numerous in patients with DAD with at least one ApoE ϵ4 allele than in those without any ApoE ϵ4 alleles.[85,86] This finding might be related to the decrease in CSF Aβ42 levels seen in these patients.

Decreased CSF Aβ42 levels have been reported in patients with non-DAD dementias,[6,30,36,41,81,84,87] bacterial meningitis in persons with DS,[88] subacute sclerosing panencephalitis,[35] Creutzfeldt–Jakob disease[48,82] and amyotrophic lateral sclerosis.[89] In 1999, Hulstaert and colleagues[35] showed that half of the patients with vascular dementia in their study sample had decreased CSF Aβ42 levels,[35] and Kanemaru and colleagues[81] found decreased Aβ42 levels in patients with Lewy body dementia. It is well known that AD pathology is a common finding in vascular dementia and Lewy body dementia.[90,91]

Combination of CSF Aβ42 and tau protein analysis in the diagnosis of Alzheimer's disease

Since measurements of any single CSF marker alone have not proved useful as a diagnostic test for DAD, a combination of different markers has been used. Tau protein has been combined with neuronal thread protein[92] and with the soluble interleukin-6 receptor complex.[93] These combinations have resulted in a specificity of 93% and 90%, respectively, and a sensitivity of 63% and 92%, respectively. However, most studies have combined measurements of CSF Aβ42 and tau protein. The sensitivity of the combination has varied from 50% to 85%. The specificity was 88–96% for controls and 58–86% for patients with non-DAD dementias. The reasons for the discrepancies may be due to differences in the patient populations, the ApoE genotype and the methodology used in the analyses. When we included only patients carrying the ApoE ϵ4 allele, the combination of tau protein and Aβ42 resulted in a sensitivity of 81% for probable diagnosis of DAD patients and 91% for neuropathologically diagnosed DAD cases.[41] The relatively high specificity of these analyses indicates that a combination of CSF Aβ42 and tau protein is a promising laboratory test for confirming the diagnosis of probable DAD.

An ideal biomarker should reflect the pathogenic processes that contribute to the progression of the disease and the neuropathological changes occurring in the brain tissue. A positive correlation with CSF Aβ levels and MMSE scores has been found in some studies[32,94,95] but not in others.[30,35] In our study,[41] neuropathologically confirmed cases with DAD had the lowest CSF Aβ42 levels, which is consistent with the finding that the lowest Aβ42 concentrations occur in patients with severe DAD.[96] Longitudinal studies indicate that CSF Aβ42 levels may remain stable for short periods (10–20 months),[30,53] but may decrease during an extended follow-up. Our three-year longitudinal study showed that CSF Aβ42 levels decrease with time in 82% of patients with DAD.[41]

A number of studies have shown that CSF Aβ40 concentrations in individuals with DAD and controls are similar.[30,39,41,97,98] However, in two studies[96,99] a decrease in CSF Aβ40 levels was found, with significant overlap between the groups. CSF Aβ40 levels showed no association with ApoE genotype in patients with DAD.

The source of Aβ in CSF and its relationship to brain pathology are not known. Some studies suggest that CSF Aβ may originate from the vessel walls. However, studies of an animal model of AD suggest that CSF Aβ is produced by neuronal cells.[100] Other studies have shown that soluble Aβ from brain parenchyma can enter CSF and blood.[101] It is also possible that part of the CSF Aβ originates from blood, since Aβ that is injected intravenously enters the brain via the blood–brain barrier.[102] However, blood is not a major source of CSF Aβ, as there is no correlation between CSF Aβ and plasma Aβ levels in patients with DAD.[98]

Aβ in plasma

Studies have shown that plasma Aβ40 and Aβ42 levels are two- to threefold higher in patients with familial DAD and with presenilin mutations than in those with sporadic DAD and controls, and that Aβ levels are approximately 100-fold lower in plasma than in CSF.[103] One study has shown that plasma Aβ40 and Aβ42 levels are similar in DAD and control groups.[104] However, our studies demonstrate that plasma Aβ40 levels are increased in individuals with DAD with the ApoE ϵ4 allele compared with those without and age-matched controls.[98] Although our results showed that mean plasma Aβ40 levels were higher in individuals with DAD than in controls, there was a considerable overlap between the two groups. Thus the measurement of plasma Aβ40 levels is not useful as a diagnostic tool for distinguishing patients with sporadic DAD from elderly nondemented controls. The finding that plasma Aβ42 levels are similar in individuals with DAD and controls is consistent with previous reports.[103,104] Discrepancies between our results and those reported by others[104] may be due to differences in patient populations.

We found increased plasma Aβ40 levels in individuals with DAD with the ApoE ϵ4 allele. However, we do not know whether these levels were present several years before the onset of probable DAD. In our recent longitudinal study of unrelated individuals, those who subsequently developed DAD had higher plasma Aβ42 levels at entry than those who remained free of dementia.[105] The results indicate that elevated plasma Aβ42 levels may be detected several years before the onset of symptoms and support the role of extracellular Aβ42 in the pathogenesis of AD. Although we found no relationship between severity of dementia and Aβ levels in the cross-sectional sample, longitudinal studies will be necessary in order to determine conclusively whether there is a relationship between plasma Aβ levels and progression of DAD. Such studies will be particularly important for determining whether modulation of plasma Aβ levels may be a useful measure of disease-modifying therapies.

The source of plasma Aβ is not known. However, it is probable that peripheral sources such as platelets are responsible for the presence of Aβ in plasma.[106,107] There are various difficulties in the measurement of Aβ in body fluids. Low concentrations of Aβ in plasma necessitate a sensitive and reliable laboratory quantitation assay. It is also known that Aβ binds to carrier proteins such as ApoE and ApoJ which are present in plasma.[108,109] It is possible that antibody epitopes of Aβ may be masked by such binding, and interfere with detection of true Aβ levels in body fluids by sandwich ELISA.

The significance of plasma Aβ levels in relation to Aβ accumulation in the brain is unclear. If plasma Aβ originates from tissues other than brain, there may not be an association between plasma Aβ levels and Aβ deposited in the brain. However, investigators have shown that Aβ and Aβ–ApoJ complexes cross the blood–brain barrier.[109] Aβ present in plasma may thus contribute to the development of Aβ deposits in the brain.

In summary, although blood is easy to obtain, it is still unclear whether there are systemic changes specific for AD, and to what extent changes in blood composition reflect pathological changes seen in the brain. CSF may be more representative of brain pathology than blood, but drawing of CSF is an invasive procedure. Further measurements of Aβ40 and Aβ42 levels in matched plasma, CSF and autopsy brain tissues, and correlation with dementia severity and ApoE genotype, are needed to increase our understanding of the significance of plasma and CSF measurement.

Aβ in Down syndrome

Down syndrome or trisomy 21 is one of the most frequent causes of mental retardation, occurring in 1 in 800 live births. Several extensive surveys of brain autopsy data of individuals with DS have reported that the neuropathology of AD is always present in individuals with DS aged 40 years or older.[110] Characteristic neuropathological changes in AD include cerebral neuritic plaques, with cores composed primarily of amyloid peptides, amyloid accumulation in meningeal and cerebral blood vessels, and neurofibrillary tangles.[111] The most likely explanation for the occurrence of these changes in the brains of individuals with DS is the presence of an extra copy of the APP gene, located on chromosome 21, which may lead to overproduction of amyloid proteins in brain and plasma. However, it is possible that chromosomal triplication induces the overexpression of other proteins which may participate in the degenerative process in DS.

Recent data showed that soluble $A\beta42$ was predominantly found in brain extracts from individuals with DS but not in controls,[112] and the levels were higher in brain extracts from individuals with DS aged 40 years or older than in those under the age of 40 years. The most likely explanation for the higher $A\beta$ levels in DS brain extracts is the presence of an extra copy of the APP gene, located on chromosome 21, which may lead to the overproduction of amyloid protein in brain and plasma. Investigators[77,113,114] have reported higher plasma levels of $A\beta40$ and $A\beta42$ in individuals with DS than in controls. However, the levels in young and old people with DS were not studied. We postulated that plasma $A\beta42$ levels would be higher in individuals with DS aged 41 years or older than in those aged 20 to 40 years.

The presence of the ApoE $\epsilon4$ allele is a significant risk factor for the development of sporadic and familial late-onset DAD.[5] Although studies have shown an association between the ApoE $\epsilon4$ allele and increased amyloid deposition in the brains of individuals with DAD, the relationship between plasma $A\beta40$ and $A\beta42$ levels and the ApoE $\epsilon4$ allele in young and old people with DS has not been examined. In this section we report the quantitation of plasma $A\beta40$ and $A\beta42$ levels in young and old people with DS and age-matched controls, and analyse the relationship with age, gender and ApoE phenotype.

Commercially synthesised $A\beta32-40$ and $A\beta33-42$ peptides (Ana Spec, San Jose, CA) were conjugated to keyhole limpet haemocyanin in phosphate-buffered saline (PBS) with 0.5% glutaraldehyde, and were then used to inoculate rabbits. The specificity of rabbit antisera R162 and R209 produced against $A\beta40$, and R165 and R226 raised against $A\beta42$ was examined in a sandwich ELISA.[115] There was a strong response of R162 and R209 with 1 ng/ml of $A\beta40$, but no detectable response with 10 ng/ml of $A\beta42$. Similarly, R165 and R226 were found to react specifically to $A\beta42$ but showed no reactivity to $A\beta40$. A Western blot test also showed that R162 and R209 were specific to $A\beta40$, and R165 and R226 were specific to $A\beta42$.[115]

Table 4.1 shows the demographic characteristics of plasma samples from DS and control groups. The groups did not differ significantly with regard to age or gender. The ApoE $\epsilon4$ allele frequency distribution was similar in individuals with DS (23.3%) and in age-matched normal controls (28.3%), consistent with reports in the literature. Plasma $A\beta40$ levels were higher in younger people with DS than in controls ($P < 0.0001$). $A\beta42$ levels in individuals with DS and in controls were similar (*see* Table 4.2). Both antisera specific to $A\beta40$ and $A\beta42$ showed similar results. Plasma $A\beta40$ levels were higher in plasma in older people with DS than in

Table 4.1 Demographic characteristics of individuals with DS and controls

Group	Mean age ± SD (years)	Gender		ApoE $\epsilon4$ allele	
		Male	Female	Positive	Negative
Young DS patients ($n = 28$)	30 ± 6	16	12	5	23
Young controls ($n = 28$)	30 ± 6	16	12	7	21
Old DS patients ($n = 32$)	51 ± 7	13	19	9	23
Old controls ($n = 32$)	51 ± 7	13	19	10	22

Table 4.2 Plasma Aβ40 and Aβ42 levels in individuals with DS and controls using two different rabbit antisera for Aβ40 and Aβ42

Group	Aβ40 (pg/ml) Median (range)		Aβ42 (pg/ml) Median (range)	
	R162	R209	R165	R226
Young DS patients	137.8 (63.8–202.8)[a]	202.0 (114.0–298.5)[a]	19.4 (10.0–27.6)	14.4 (7.0–30.5)
Young controls	75.0 (40.0–121.2)	123.0 (75.9–179.7)	17.3 (8.5–28.7)	14.6 (4.9–24.4)
Old DS patients	122.4 (57.7–267.2)[b]	190.7 (94.3–310.0)[b]	21.0 (14.8–56.3)[c]	19.6 (7.3–41.8)[c]
Old controls	79.0 (36.7–123.3)	120.3 (54.5–184.3)	16.2 (11.3–27.5)	13.9 (6.5–29.2)

[a] Significant differences in Aβ40 levels compared with young controls ($P < 0.0001$).
[b] Significant differences in Aβ40 levels compared with old controls ($P < 0.0001$).
[c] Significant differences in Aβ42 levels compared with old controls using R165 ($P < 0.012$) and using R226 ($P < 0.006$).

controls ($P < 0.0001$). Aβ42 levels were also higher in people with DS than in controls ($P < 0.012$ with R165, and $P < 0.006$ with R226) (*see* Table 4.2).

Plasma Aβ40 and Aβ42 levels in young and old controls were similar. Aβ40 levels in younger patients with DS and in older patients with DS were similar. However, Aβ42 levels were higher in older patients with DS than in younger patients with DS ($P < 0.04$) with R226, but did not reach the level of significance with R165 ($P < 0.09$).

There was no correlation between age and Aβ40 or Aβ42 levels in younger patients with DS, and young or old controls. However, there was a significant correlation between age and Aβ40 levels for older patients with DS ($r = 0.42$, $P < 0.015$), and between age and Aβ42 levels for older patients with DS ($r = 0.41$, $P < 0.017$ with R226, but not with R165). There was no significant relationship between gender and Aβ40 or Aβ42 levels in any of the four groups, and there was no association of Aβ40 or Aβ42 levels with the ApoE ϵ4 allele in either the DS or control groups.

There was a significant association between Aβ40 and Aβ42 levels for young controls ($r = 0.657$, $P < 0.001$), younger patients with DS ($r = 0.558$, $P < 0.002$), old controls ($r = 0.38$, $P < 0.028$ with R162 and R165 but not with R209 and R226) and older patients with DS ($r = 0.597$, $P < 0.001$ with R209 and R226 but not with R162 and R165).

Our results showed significantly higher plasma levels of Aβ40 and Aβ42 in older patients with DS than in older controls by using two different rabbit antibodies specific for Aβ40 and Aβ42, respectively, and higher plasma levels of Aβ42 in older patients with DS than in younger patients with DS when R226 was employed. These findings are consistent with the higher plasma Aβ40 and Aβ42 levels seen in patients with DAD associated with APP, presenilin 1 or presenilin 2 mutations.[103] However, the results differ from those for individuals with sporadic DAD, where plasma Aβ42 levels were similar to those in non-demented age-matched controls.[98] Since there are no commercially available ELISA kits to quantitate low levels of plasma Aβ40 and Aβ42, investigators have developed ELISA using mouse monoclonal or rabbit antibodies specific to Aβ40 and Aβ42, respectively.[77,113,114] Although in the present study plasma levels of Aβ40 and Aβ42 were somewhat different from one specific antibody to another (*see* Table 4.2), our overall results were similar. The reason for the discrepancy is not clear, but it could result from differences in the affinity of specific rabbit Aβ antiserum, and the purity, conformation or solubilisation of Aβ40 and Aβ42 peptides used as standards.

The higher plasma Aβ40 levels seen in younger and older patients with DS are consistent with recent observations of the presence of intraneuronal Aβ40 staining in the hippocampus and cerebral cortex of the brain from patients with DS.[116,117] The higher plasma Aβ42 levels in older patients with DS compared with old controls or young DS patients suggests that Aβ42 levels are selectively increased in plasma with the development of AD neuropathology in this group. The significant increase in Aβ42 levels in older patients with DS compared with controls is consistent with the results of recent immunocytochemical studies, which showed increased deposition of extracellular Aβ and formation of Aβ42-positive plaques in the brains of patients with DS,[116,117] and higher levels of soluble Aβ42 levels in DS brain extracts than in controls.[112] The intracellular accumulation of Aβ in the brains of individuals with DS may be due to over-expression of the APP gene–dose effect on APP. However, deposition of Aβ42 in brain tissues is not likely to result directly from increased plasma Aβ42 levels. Investigators have suggested that some Aβ in brain parenchyma can be eliminated through the perivascular spaces and may influence Aβ levels in blood.[118] However, studies have shown that anti-Aβ immunoreactivity in blood is associated with platelets.[106]

We found no relationship between the ApoE ϵ4 allele and Aβ40 or Aβ42 levels in either group, consistent with previous reports.[113] However, our preliminary studies[119] showed that plasma Aβ42 levels were higher in DS patients with dementia with the ApoE ϵ4 allele than in those without it. In the present study the number of individuals with DS with the ApoE ϵ4 allele is small, so further studies employing larger samples are essential to confirm the relationship of ApoE alleles to Aβ40 and Aβ42 levels in demented and non-demented adults with DS. Longitudinal measurements of plasma Aβ40 and Aβ42 levels in individuals with DS aged 40 years or older, and correlation with cognitive function and behaviour analysis, might be useful for predicting the risk of developing dementia in individuals with DS.

Tau protein in Down syndrome

It has been shown that tau protein levels are higher in brains from individuals with DS and in people from the general population with DAD than in those from elderly non-demented controls or patients with other neurological diseases.[120] Recent studies have shown the presence of tau-like protein in plasma from individuals with DAD and controls. We measured plasma tau-like protein levels from individuals with DS, non-DS age-matched controls, non-DS individuals with intellectual disability (ID), individuals with DAD and elderly non-demented controls.

Plasma tau-like protein levels were quantitated using a double monoclonal antibody-based sandwich ELISA (Innotest hTau antigen kit, Innogenetics NV, Belgium) according to the manufacturer's instructions.[33] The assay includes antisera which recognise both phosphorylated and non-phosphorylated epitopes of tau. The detection limit for plasma tau-like protein was 35 pg/ml. The mean coefficient of intra-assay variation was 8.7% and the mean coefficient of intra-assay variation was 13.1%. The groups were compared with each constituent using the Mann–Whitney or Kruskal–Wallis one-way analysis of variance with a Bonferroni correction for multiple comparisons. Pearson's correlation with Bonferroni correction was used to analyse the relationship between the variables.

Table 4.3 shows the demographic characteristics of the individuals with DS, ID and DAD and the controls who were included in the study. The DS patients, non-DS age-matched normal controls and non-DS patients with ID did not differ significantly with regard to age or gender. Similarly, the DAD and non-demented elderly control groups showed no significant difference with regard to age or gender. The ApoE frequencies were similar in individuals with DS (27.5%) and age-matched controls (32.5%). As expected, the ApoE ϵ4 allele frequencies were higher in individuals with DAD (68%) than in any other group.

Tau-like protein levels were detected in 22 out of 40 DS patients, 4 of 40 non-DS age-matched controls, 1 of 18 non-DS patients with ID, none of 25 patients with DAD and 1 of 24 elderly non-demented controls (*see* Figure 4.1). The levels were significantly higher in DS patients than in the control, ID and DAD groups ($P < 0.0001$) (*see* Figure 4.1). However, the levels were similar among non-DS normal controls and the ID, DAD and non-demented elderly control groups. There was no significant association between tau-like protein levels and age or gender in any of the five groups. The levels did not differ significantly between patients with DS with the ApoE ϵ4 allele (median, 136.2 pg/ml; range, 53–1596 pg/ml) and in those without the allele (median, 71.8 pg/ml; range, < 35–4306 pg/ml) ($P = 0.74$).

Comparative studies of individuals with DS and those with DAD in the general population have shown that the development of pathological changes in DS does

Table 4.3 Plasma tau-like protein levels in DS patients, non-DS patients with ID, AD patients and controls

Group	Age (years) Median (range)	Gender		ApoE ϵ4 allele	
		Male	Female	Positive	Negative
DS patients (*n* = 40)	45.5 (31–70)	18	22	11	29
Non-DS age-matched controls (*n* = 40)	44.0 (31–71)	16	24	13	27
Non-DS patients with ID (*n* = 18)	45.5 (26–91)	8	10	6	12
AD patients (*n* = 25)	74.0 (55–99)	13	12	17	8
Elderly non-demented controls (*n* = 24)	69.5 (54–79)	11	13	7	17

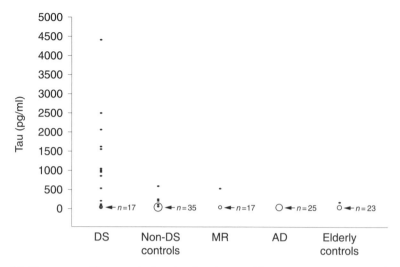

Figure 4.1 Plasma tau-like protein levels of patients with DS, non-DS age-matched normal controls, non-DS mentally retarded (MR) individuals, patients with AD and elderly non-demented controls.

not parallel that in adults with DAD in the general population.[121,122] For example, individuals with DS have higher NFT densities than patients with DAD, and the concentration of protease-resistant particulate tau protein is threefold higher in brains from individuals with DS than in those from the general population with DAD. Tau-like protein was not detected in about half of DS plasma examined by ELISA. This finding is not unusual, as previous studies[123] have shown that there is substantial variation in neurofibrillary pathology in brains from individuals with DS.

A number of studies have shown that CSF tau levels are increased in patients with DAD compared with controls, and these levels might be useful for supporting the diagnosis of probable DAD.[28,33,40] In contrast, a recent report showed that CSF tau levels were not increased in 11 patients with DS compared with adults with DAD. The reason for the discrepancy is unclear apart from the fact that the sample size was too small. Further studies using a larger number of patients with DS are necessary in order to clarify these controversial findings.

It is still not known to what extent changes in blood composition reflect pathological changes seen in the brain. CSF may be more representative of brain pathology than blood. However, lumbar puncture is an invasive procedure. Further measurements of tau-like protein levels in matched plasma and autopsy brain tissues and correlation with the ApoE genotype and dementia severity are needed to increase our understanding of the significance of plasma tau-like protein in individuals with DS. Longitudinal measurements of plasma tau-like protein levels in ageing individuals with DS are essential to determine whether this assay is potentially useful for predicting the risk of developing of DAD and as a peripheral marker of brain pathology to monitor severity of dementia.

Problems and limitations in the search for a biomarker for Alzheimer's disease

The Consensus Group suggests that an 'ideal' biomarker should have a sensitivity and specificity of more than 80% for correct identification of non-DAD dementias.[124] A core criterion for a reliable biomarker is that it should reflect a fundamental feature of AD pathophysiology. Moreover, in addition to its value as a tool for accurate differential diagnosis, an ideal biomarker for AD should have the potential to track disease progression, and it needs to be reliable, reproducible, non-invasive, simple to perform and inexpensive.

Selection of patient material is critical and varies in different studies. In general, most studies have included a small number of patients with DAD and non-demented controls, and lacked appropriate controls, such as patients with other types of dementia. Since the studies have been conducted using living patients with probable DAD, the classification of the patients is of utmost importance. Although the diagnosis of probable DAD can be made accurately in over 85% of cases using the NINCDS–ADRDA criteria,[12] it is difficult to rule out the presence of underlying AD pathology in control groups. In addition, patients with other dementias, such as vascular dementia or Lewy body dementia, often have coexisting AD neuropathology. This would explain the limited specificity of CSF tau protein or $A\beta$ measurements for discriminating between patients with DAD and those with non-DAD dementias.

The measured levels of CSF $A\beta40$ and $A\beta42$ differed from one research laboratory to another. These conflicting results may be due to differences in the affinity of specific $A\beta$ antisera, and in the purity and solubilisation of peptides used as standards. In addition to the differences in the ELISA methods, conflicting data could also be due to differences in sample collection and storage conditions. It has been reported that measured $A\beta$ levels decrease over time, even if the CSF is frozen.[73] Multiple freezing and thawing of CSF could also result in the loss of $A\beta$. Several studies have shown that $A\beta$ levels are lower in CSF collected in glass or polystyrene tubes than in polypropylene ones.

Finally, the usefulness of a putative marker is related to the role of a given substance in the aetiology and pathogenesis of the disease. Alzheimer's disease is a complex, genetically and aetiologically heterogeneous disorder with a stage-specific pattern of neuropathological changes rather than a single abnormality in the brain. The biochemical processes that contribute to the pathogenesis and progression of DAD are numerous and poorly understood, and may be different in patients with familial and sporadic DAD or in those with early-onset and late-onset disease. Thus it is possible that no single diagnostic marker will be found for different forms of AD. For example, the measurement of $A\beta$ levels in CSF or fibroblast culture medium may help to identify affected individuals with familial DAD associated with APP mutations, but its usefulness in other forms of AD is unknown. Although recent studies[34] have recommended the measurement of CSF $A\beta42$ levels and microtubule-associated tau protein concentrations in order to support the diagnosis of AD, this assay is not widely used because it requires a lumbar puncture to be performed. It is likely that some combination of distinct markers (preferably from plasma or serum) with quantitative neuroimaging, used in conjunction with clinical and neurobehavioural assessments, will be necessary in order to diagnose probable DAD, and to monitor the progression of the disease.[125]

Conclusion

Alzheimer's disease is a neurodegenerative condition that affects cognition, behaviour and function. The aetiology of the disease is unknown, but the primary risk factors for DAD are ageing and family history. Neurofibrillary tangles and amyloid-bearing neuritic plaques in the limbic and cerebral cortices are the characteristic neuropathological lesions in the brains of patients with DAD. The NFT are composed mainly of hyperphosphorylated tau protein, whereas the major component of the neuritic plaques is Aβ. The clinical diagnosis of probable DAD is based on history, physical examination, neuropsychological testing, laboratory studies and neuroimaging techniques. However, there is no laboratory marker to support the diagnosis of definite DAD or monitoring of the progression of the disease. Several biochemical markers related to neuropathology have been identified in CSF. This chapter has described the studies of CSF or blood levels of tau protein, and Aβ, in patients with AD and in age-matched non-demented controls. Due to the heterogeneity and complex nature of the disease, it is highly unlikely that a single marker specific for AD will be found. However, a panel of biomarkers may help to discriminate different subgroups of AD with distinct genetic backgrounds.

Down syndrome is one of the most frequent causes of ID, occurring in 1 in 800 live births. Several surveys of brain autopsy data of DS patients have reported that the neuropathology of AD is present in individuals with DS aged 40 years or older. The pathological changes include the presence of neuritic plaques and neurofibrillary tangles. The core protein of neuritic plaques is Aβ. There are two major forms of Aβ, namely Aβ40 and Aβ42. The latter is predominantly found in brain extracts from individuals with DS. We have recently quantitated the levels of Aβ40 and Aβ42 in blood from young (20–40 years of age) and older (41–65 years) patients with DS. We found that Aβ42 levels were similar in young people with DS and age-matched normal controls. However, the levels were higher in older people with DS than in age-matched normal controls. The higher levels of Aβ42 in older people with DS suggest that the concentration of Aβ42 is selectively increased in blood during the development of AD pathology. Longitudinal measurements of Aβ levels in individuals with DS over the age of 40 years, and correlation with cognitive function and behaviour analysis, might be useful for predicting the early signs of dementia in individuals with DS and for monitoring the severity of dementia in this population.

References

1 Richards SS and Hendrie HC (1999) Diagnosis, management and treatment of Alzheimer disease. *Arch Intern Med.* **159**: 789–98.
2 Small GW, Rabins PV, Barry PP *et al.* (1999) Diagnosis and treatment of Alzheimer disease and related disorders. Consensus Statement of the American Association for Geriatric Psychiatry, the Alzheimer's Association and the American Geriatrics Society. *JAMA.* **278**: 1363–71.
3 Tanzi RE (1999) A genetic dichotomy model for the inheritance of Alzheimer disease and common age-related disorders. *J Clin Invest.* **104**: 1175–9.

4 Corder EH, Saunders AM, Strittmatter WJ *et al.* (1993) Gene dose of apolipoprotein E type 4 allele and the risk of Alzheimer disease in late-onset families. *Science.* **261:** 921–3.

5 Saunders AM, Strittmatter WJ, Schemechel D *et al.* (1993) Association of apolipoprotein E allele ϵ4 with late-onset familial and sporadic Alzheimer disease. *Neurology.* **43:** 1467–72.

6 Selkoe D (1994) Normal and abnormal biology of the β-amyloid precursor protein. *Annu Rev Neurosci.* **17:** 489–517.

7 Wisniewski HM and Wegiel J (1995) The neuropathology of Alzheimer's disease. *Neuroimaging Clin North Am.* **5:** 45–57.

8 Hass C, Scholossmacher MG, Hung A-Y *et al.* (1992) Amyloid-2-peptide is produced by cultured cells during normal metabolism. *Nature.* **359:** 322–6.

9 Mehta PD, Kim KS and Wisniewski HM (1997) ELISA as a laboratory test to aid the diagnosis of Alzheimer's disease. *Techniques Diagn Pathol.* **2:** 99–112.

10 Seubert P, Vigo-Pelfrey C, Esch F *et al.* (1992) Isolation and quantitation of soluble Alzheimer's Aβ-peptide from biological fluids. *Nature.* **359:** 325–7.

11 Younkin SG (1995) Evidence that Aβ42 is the real culprit in Alzheimer disease. *Ann Neurol.* **37:** 287–8.

12 McKhann G, Drachman D, Folstien M *et al.* (1984) Clinical diagnosis of Alzheimer disease: report of the NINCDS–ADRDA work group under the auspices of the Department of Health and Human Services Task Force on Alzheimer Disease. *Neurology.* **34:** 939–44.

13 Petersen RC, Smith GE, Waring SC *et al.* (1999) Mild cognitive impairment: clinical characterization and outcome. *Arch Neurol.* **56:** 303–8.

14 Segal MB (1993) Extracellular and cerebrospinal fluids. *J Inherit Metab Dis.* **16:** 617–38.

15 Goedert M, Spillantini MG, Potier MC *et al.* (1989) Cloning and sequencing of the cDNA encoding an isoform of microtubule-associated protein tau containing four tandem repeats: differential expression of tau protein mRNAs in human brain. *EMBO J.* **8:** 393–9.

16 Kosik KS, Crandall JE, Mufson EJ *et al.* (1989) Tau *in situ* hybridization in normal and Alzheimer brain: localization in the somatodendritic compartment. *Ann Neurol.* **26:** 352–61.

17 Papasozomenos SC (1989) Tau protein immunoreactivity in dementia of the Alzheimer type. I. Morphology, evolution, distribution and pathogenetic implications. *Lab Invest.* **60:** 123–37.

18 LoPresti P, Szuchet S, Papasozomenos SC *et al.* (1995) Functional implications for the microtubule-associated protein tau: localization in oligodendrocytes. *Proc Natl Acad Sci USA.* **92:** 10369–73.

19 Matsuyama SS and Bondareff W (1994) Tau-like immunoreactivity in Alzheimer and control skin fibroblasts. *J Neurosci Res.* **39:** 519–24.

20 Arai H, Terajima M, Miura M *et al.* (1995) Tau in cerebrospinal fluid: a potential diagnostic marker in Alzheimer's disease. *Ann Neurol.* **38:** 649–52.

21 Ishiguro K, Ohno H, Arai H *et al.* (1999) Phosphorylated tau in human cerebrospinal fluid is a diagnostic marker for Alzheimer's disease. *Neurosci Lett.* **270:** 91–4.

22 Johnson GV, Seubert P, Cox TM *et al.* (1997) The tau protein in human cerebrospinal fluid in Alzheimer's disease consists of proteolytically derived fragments. *J Neurochem.* **68:** 430–3.

23 Vigo-Pelfrey C, Seubert P, Barbour R *et al.* (1995) Elevation of microtubule-associated protein tau in the cerebrospinal fluid of patients with Alzheimer's disease. *Neurology.* **45:** 788–93.

24 Wolozin B and Davies P (1987) Alzheimer-related neuronal protein A68: specificity and distribution. *Ann Neurol.* **22:** 521–6.

25 Zemlan FP, Rosenberg WS, Luebbe PA *et al.* (1999) Quantification of axonal damage in traumatic brain injury: affinity purification and characterization of cerebrospinal fluid tau proteins. *J Neurochem.* **72:** 741–50.

26 Sussmuth SD, Reiber H and Tumani H (2001) Tau protein in cerebrospinal fluid (CSF): a blood–CSF barrier-related evaluation in patients with various neurological diseases. *Neurosci Lett.* **300:** 95–8.

27 Tapiola T, Overmyer M, Lehtovirta M *et al.* (1997) The level of cerebrospinal fluid tau correlates with neurofibrillary tangles in Alzheimer's disease. *Neuroreport.* **8:** 3961–3.

28 Blennow K, Wallin A, Agren H *et al.* (1995) Tau protein in cerebrospinal fluid: a biochemical marker for axonal degeneration in Alzheimer disease? *Mol Chem Neuropathol.* **26:** 231–45.

29 Blomberg M, Jensen M, Basun H *et al.* (2001) Cerebrospinal fluid tau levels increase with age in healthy individuals. *Dement Geriatr Cogn Disord.* **12:** 127–32.

30 Kanai M, Matsubara E, Isoe K *et al.* (1998) Longitudinal study of cerebrospinal fluid levels of tau, Aβ 1–40, and Aβ 1–42(43) in Alzheimer's disease: a study in Japan. *Ann Neurol.* **44:** 17–26.

31 Sjogren M, Vanderstichele H, Agren H *et al.* (2001) Tau and Aβ42 in cerebrospinal fluid from healthy adults 21–93 years of age: establishment of reference values. *Clin Chem.* **47:** 1776–81.

32 Galasko D, Chang L, Motter R *et al.* (1998) High cerebrospinal fluid tau and low amyloid β42 levels in the clinical diagnosis of Alzheimer disease and relation to apolipoprotein E genotype. *Arch Neurol.* **55:** 937–45.

33 Vandermeeren M, Mercken M, Vanmechelen E *et al.* (1993) Detection of tau proteins in normal and Alzheimer's disease cerebrospinal fluid with a sensitive sandwich enzyme-linked immunosorbent assay. *J Neurochem.* **61:** 1828–34.

34 Andreasen N, Minthon L, Davidsson P *et al.* (2001) Evaluation for CSF-tau and CSF-Aβ42 as diagnostic markers for Alzheimer disease in clinical practice. *Arch Neurol.* **58:** 373–9.

35 Hulstaert F, Blennow K, Ivanoiu A *et al.* (1999) Improved discrimination of AD patients using beta-amyloid (1–42) and tau levels in CSF. *Neurology.* **52:** 1555–62.

36 Motter R, Vigo-Pelfrey C, Khodolenko D *et al.* (1995) Reduction of beta-amyloid peptide 42 in the cerebrospinal fluid of patients with Alzheimer's disease. *Ann Neurol.* **38:** 643–8.

37 Munroe WA, Southwick PC, Chang L *et al.* (1995) Tau protein in cerebrospinal fluid as an aid in the diagnosis of Alzheimer's disease. *Ann Clin Lab Sci.* **25:** 207–17.

38 Nishimura T, Takeda M, Nakamura Y *et al.* (1998) Basic and clinical studies on the measurement of tau protein in cerebrospinal fluid as a biological marker for Alzheimer's disease and related disorders: multicenter study in Japan. *Methods Find Exp Clin Pharmacol.* **20:** 227–35.

39 Shoji M, Matsubara E, Kanai M *et al.* (1998) Combination assay of CSF tau, Aβ1–40 and Aβ1–42(43) as a biochemical marker of Alzheimer's disease. *J Neurol Sci.* **158:** 134–40.

40 Tapiola T, Lehtovirta M, Ramberg J *et al.* (2000) CSF tau is related to apoE genotype in early Alzheimer's disease. *Neurology.* **50:** 169–74.

41 Tapiola T, Pirttil T, Mehta PD *et al.* (2000) Relationship between apoE genotype and CSF β-amyloid (1–42) and tau in patients with probable and definite Alzheimer's disease. *Neurobiol Aging.* **21:** 735–40.

42 Golombowski S, Muller-Spahn F, Romig H *et al.* (1997) Dependence of cerebrospinal fluid tau protein levels on apolipoprotein E4 allele frequency in patients with Alzheimer's disease. *Neurosci Lett.* **225:** 213–15.

43 Molina L, Touchon J, Herpe M *et al.* (1999) Tau and apoE in CSF: potential aid for discriminating Alzheimer's disease from other dementias. *Neuroreport.* **10:** 3491–5.

44 Andreasen N, Minthon L, Clarberg A *et al.* (1999) Sensitivity, specificity and stability of CSF-tau in AD in a community-based patient sample. *Neurology.* **53:** 1488–94.

45 Arai H, Morikawa Y, Higuchi M *et al.* (1976) Cerebrospinal fluid tau levels in neurodegenerative diseases with distinct tau-related pathology. *Biochem Biophys Res Commun.* **236:** 262–4.

46 Kurz A, Riemenschneider M, Buch K *et al.* (1998) Tau protein in cerebrospinal fluid is significantly increased at the earliest clinical stage of Alzheimer disease. *Alzheimer Dis Assoc Disord.* **12:** 372–7.

47 Sunderland T, Wolozin B, Galasko D *et al.* (1999) Longitudinal stability of CSF tau levels in Alzheimer patients. *Biol Psychiatry.* **46:** 750–5.

48 Kapaki E, Kilidireas K, Paraskevas GP *et al.* (2001) Highly increased CSF tau protein and decreased β-amyloid (1–42) in sporadic CJD: a discrimination from Alzheimer's disease? *J Neurol Neurosurg Psychiatry.* **71:** 401–3.

49 Otto M, Wiltfang J, Cepek L *et al.* (2002) Tau protein and 14–3–3 protein in the differential diagnosis of Creutzfeldt–Jakob disease. *Neurology.* **58:** 192–7.

50 Hesse C, Rosengren L, Andreasen N *et al.* (2001) Transient increase in total tau but not phospho-tau in human cerebrospinal fluid after stroke. *Neurosci Lett.* **297:** 187–90.

51 Galasko D, Clark C, Chang L *et al.* (1997) Assessment of CSF levels of tau protein in mildly demented patients with Alzheimer's disease. *Neurology.* **48:** 632–5.

52 Riemenschneider M, Buch K, Schmolke M *et al.* (1996) Cerebrospinal protein tau is elevated in early Alzheimer's disease. *Neurosci Lett.* **212:** 209–11.

53 Andreasen N, Minthon L, Vanmechelen E *et al.* (1999) Cerebrospinal fluid tau and Aβ42 as predictors of development of Alzheimer's disease in patients with mild cognitive impairment. *Neurosci Lett.* **273:** 5–8.

54 Galasko D, Chang L, Motter R *et al.* (1998) High cerebrospinal fluid tau and low amyloid β42 levels in the clinical diagnosis of Alzheimer's disease and relation to apolipoprotein E genotype. *Arch Neurol.* **55:** 937–45.

55 Mecocci P, Cherubini A, Bregnocchi M *et al.* (1998) Tau protein in cerebrospinal fluid: a new diagnostic and prognostic marker in Alzheimer disease? *Alzheimer Dis Assoc Disord.* **12:** 211–14.

56 Isoe K, Urakami K, Shimomura T *et al.* (1996) Tau proteins in cerebrospinal fluid from patients with Alzheimer's disease: a longitudinal study. *Dementia.* **7:** 175–6.

57 Andreasen N, Vanmechelen E, Van De Voorde A *et al.* (1998) Cerebrospinal fluid tau protein as a biochemical marker for Alzheimer's disease: a community-based follow-up study. *J Neurol Neurosurg Psychiatry.* **64:** 298–305.

58 Tapiola T, Pirttil T, Mikkonen M *et al.* (2000) Three-year follow-up of cerebrospinal fluid tau, β-amyloid 42 and 40 concentrations in Alzheimer's disease. *Neurosci Lett.* **280:** 119–22.

59 Braak H and Braak E (1995) Staging of Alzheimer's disease-related neurofibrillary changes. *Neurobiol Aging.* **16:** 271–8.

60 Blennow K, Vanmechelen E and Hampel H (2001) CSF total tau, Aβ 1–42 and phosphorylated tau protein as biomarkers for Alzheimer's disease. *Mol Neurobiol.* **24:** 87–97.

61 Kohnken R, Buerger K, Zinkowski R *et al.* (2000) Detection of tau phosphorylated at threonine 231 in cerebrospinal fluid of Alzheimer's disease patients. *Neurosci Lett.* **287:** 187–90.

62 Burger K, Teipel SJ, Zinkowski R *et al.* (2002) CSF tau protein phosphorylated at threonine 231 correlates with cognitive decline in MCI subjects. *Neurology.* **59:** 627–9.

63 Burger K, Zinkowski R, Teipel SJ *et al.* (2003) Differentiation of geriatric major depression from Alzheimer's disease with CSF tau protein phosphorylated at threonine 231. *Am J Psychiatry.* **160:** 376–9.

64 Itoh N, Arai H, Urakami K *et al.* (2001) Large-scale, multicenter study of cerebrospinal fluid tau protein phosphorylated at serine 199 for the antemortem diagnosis of Alzheimer's disease. *Ann Neurol.* **50:** 150–6.

65 Hampel H, Burger K, Kohnken R et al. (2001) Tracking of Alzheimer's disease progression with cerebrospinal fluid tau protein phosphorylated at threonine 231. *Ann Neurol.* **49:** 545–6.

66 De Leon MJ, Segal CY, Tarshish CY et al. (2002) Longitudinal CSF tau load increases in mild cognitive impairment. *Neurosci Lett.* **333:** 183–6.

67 Lubke U, Six J, Villanova A et al. (1994) Microtubule-associated protein tau epitopes are present in fiber lesions in diverse muscle disorders. *Am J Pathol.* **145:** 175–88.

68 Ingelson M, Blomberg M, Benedikz E et al. (1999) Tau immunoreactivity detected in human plasma, but not increased in Alzheimer disease. *Dement Geriatr Cogn Disord.* **10:** 442–5.

69 Gravina SA, Libin H, Eckman CB et al. (1995) Amyloid β protein (Aβ) in Alzheimer's disease brain: biochemical and immunocytochemical analysis with antibodies specific for forms of Aβ40 and Aβ42(43). *J Biol Chem.* **270:** 7013–16.

70 Pirttila T, Kim KS, Mehta PD et al. (1994) Soluble amyloid beta-protein in the cerebrospinal fluid from patients with Alzheimer's disease, vascular dementia and controls. *J Neurol Sci.* **127:** 90–5.

71 Nakamura T, Shoji M, Harigaya Y et al. (1994) Amyloid β protein levels in cerebrospinal fluid are elevated in early-onset Alzheimer's disease. *Ann Neurol.* **36:** 903–11.

72 Nitsch RM, Rebeck GW, Deng M et al. (1995) Cerebrospinal fluid levels of amyloid β protein in Alzheimer's disease: inverse correlation with severity of dementia and effect of apolipoprotein E genotype. *Ann Neurol.* **37:** 512–18.

73 Southwick PC, Yamagata SK, Echols CL et al. (1996) Assessment of amyloid beta protein in cerebrospinal fluid as an aid in the diagnosis of Alzheimer's disease. *J Neurochem.* **66:** 259–65.

74 Van Gool WA, Kuiper MA, Walstra GJM et al. (1995) Concentrations of amyloid β protein in cerebrospinal fluid of patients with Alzheimer's disease. *Ann Neurol.* **37:** 277–9.

75 Pirttila T, Mehta PD, Soininen H et al. (1996) Cerebrospinal fluid concentrations of soluble amyloid beta-protein and apolipoprotein E in patients with Alzheimer's disease: correlations with amyloid load in the brain. *Arch Neurol.* **53:** 189–93.

76 Jensen M, Hatmann T, Engvall B et al. (2000) Quantification of Alzheimer amyloid β peptides ending at residues 40 and 42 by novel ELISA systems. *Mol Med.* **6:** 291–302.

77 Mehta PD, Dalton AJ, Mehta SP et al. (1998) Increased plasma amyloid beta protein 1–42 levels in Down syndrome. *Neurosci Lett.* **241:** 13–16.

78 Suzuki N, Cheung TT, Cai XD et al. (1994) An increased percentage of long amyloid beta protein secreted by familial amyloid beta protein precursor (beta APP717) mutants. *Science.* **264:** 1336–40.

79 Vanderstichele H, Van Kerschaver E, Hesse C et al. (2000) Standardization of measurement of β-amyloid(1–42) in cerebrospinal fluid and plasma. *Int J Exp Clin Invest.* **7:** 245–58.

80 Andreasen M, Hesse C, Davidsson P et al. (1999) Cerebrospinal fluid beta-amyloid(1–42) in Alzheimer disease: differences between early- and late-onset Alzheimer disease and stability during the course of disease. *Arch Neurol.* **56:** 673–80.

81 Kanemaru K, Kameda N and Yamanouchi H (2000) Decreased CSF amyloid β42 and normal tau levels in dementia with Lewy bodies. *Neurology.* **54:** 1875–6.

82 Otto M, Esselmann H, Schulz-Shaeffer W et al. (2000). Decreased beta-amyloid 1–42 in cerebrospinal fluid of patients with Creutzfeldt–Jakob disease. *Neurology.* **54:** 1099–102.

83 Riemenschneider M, Schmolke M, Lautenschlager N et al. (2000) Cerebrospinal beta-amyloid (1–42) in early Alzheimer's disease: association with apolipoprotein E genotype and cognitive decline. *Neurosci Lett.* **284:** 85–8.

84 Sjogren M, Minthon L, Davidsson P et al. (2000) CSF levels of tau, β-amyloid 1–42 and GAP-43 in frontotemporal dementia, other types of dementia and normal aging. *J Neural Transm.* **107:** 563–79.

85 Rebeck GW, Reiter JS, Strickland DK *et al.* (1993) Apolipoprotein E in sporadic Alzheimer's disease: allelic variation and receptor interactions. *Neuron.* 11: 575–80.

86 Schmechel DE, Saunders AM, Strittmatter WJ *et al.* (1993) Increased amyloid beta-peptide deposition in cerebral cortex as a consequence of apolipoprotein E genotype in late-onset Alzheimer disease. *Proc Natl Acad Sci USA.* 90: 9649–53.

87 Tamaoka A, Sawamura N, Fukushima T *et al.* (1997) Amyloid beta protein 42(43) in cerebrospinal fluid of patients with Alzheimer's disease. *J Neurol Sci.* 148: 41–5.

88 Tamaoka A, Sekijima Y, Matsuno S *et al.* (1999) Amyloid beta protein species in cerebrospinal fluid and in brain from patients with Down's syndrome. *Ann Neurol.* 46: 933.

89 Sjogren M, Davidsson P, Wallin A *et al.* (2002) Decreased CSF beta-amyloid 42 in Alzheimer's disease and amyotrophic lateral sclerosis may reflect mismetabolism of beta-amyloid-induced disparate mechanisms. *Dement Geriatr Cogn Disord.* 13: 112–18.

90 Galasko D, Hansen LA, Katzman R *et al.* (1994) Clinical–neuropathological correlations in Alzheimer's disease and related dementias. *Arch Neurol.* 51: 888–95.

91 Londos E, Passant U, Gustafson L *et al.* (2001) Neuropathological correlates to clinically defined dementia with Lewy bodies. *Int J Geriatr Psychiatry.* 16: 667–9.

92 Kahle PJ, Jakewec M, Teipel SJ *et al.* (2000) Combined assessment of tau and neuronal thread protein in Alzheimer's disease CSF. *Neurology.* 54: 1498–504.

93 Hampel H, Teipel SJ, Padberg F *et al.* (1999) Discriminant power of combined cerebrospinal fluid tau protein and of the soluble interleukin-6 receptor complex in the diagnosis of Alzheimer's disease. *Brain Res.* 823: 104–12.

94 Maruyama M, Arai H, Sugita M *et al.* (2001) Cerebrospinal fluid amyloid β1–42 levels in the mild cognitive impairment stage of Alzheimer's disease. *Exp Neurol.* 172: 433–6.

95 Samuels SC, Silverman JM, Marin DB *et al.* (1999) CSF beta-amyloid, cognition, and ApoE genotype in Alzheimer's disease. *Neurology.* 52: 547–51.

96 Jensen M, Schroder J, Blomberg M *et al.* (1999) Cerebrospinal fluid A beta42 is increased early in sporadic Alzheimer's disease and declines with disease progression. *Ann Neurol.* 45: 504–11.

97 Ida N, Hartmann T, Pantel J *et al.* (1996) Analysis of heterogeneous A4 peptides in human cerebrospinal fluid and blood by a newly developed sensitive Western blot assay. *J Biol Chem.* 271: 908–14.

98 Mehta PD, Pirttil T, Mehta SP *et al.* (2000) Plasma and cerebrospinal fluid levels of amyloid beta proteins 1–40 and 1–42 in Alzheimer disease. *Arch Neurol.* 57: 100–5.

99 Schroder J, Pantel J, Ida N *et al.* (1997) Cerebral changes and cerebrospinal fluid beta-amyloid in Alzheimer's disease: a study with quantitative magnetic resonance imaging. *Mol Psychiatry.* 2: 505–7.

100 Calhoun M, Burgermeister P, Phinney A *et al.* (1999) Neuronal overexpression of mutant amyloid precursor protein results in prominent deposition of cerebrovascular amyloid. *Proc Natl Acad Sci USA.* 96: 14088–93.

101 Pluta R, Barcikowska M, Misicka A *et al.* (1999) Ischemic rats as a model in the study of the neurobiological role of human beta-amyloid peptide. Time-dependent disappearing diffuse amyloid plaques in brain. *Neuroreport.* 10: 3615–19.

102 Maness LM, Banks WA, Podlisny MB *et al.* (1994) Passage of human amyloid beta-protein 1–40 across the murine blood–brain barrier. *Life Sci.* 55: 1643–50.

103 Scheuner D, Eckman C, Jensen M *et al.* (1996) Secreted amyloid beta-protein similar to that in the senile plaques of Alzheimer's disease is increased *in vivo* by the presenilin 1 and 2 and APP mutations linked to familial Alzheimer's disease. *Nat Med.* 2: 864–70.

104 Tamaoka A, Fukushima T, Sawamura N *et al.* (1996) Amyloid beta protein in plasma from patients with sporadic Alzheimer's disease. *J Neurol Sci.* 141: 65–8.

105 Mayeux R, Tang MX, Jacobs DM *et al.* (1999) Plasma amyloid beta-peptide 1–42 and incipient Alzheimer's disease. *Ann Neurol.* 46: 412–16.

106 Chen M, Inestrosa NC, Ross GS *et al.* (1995) Platelets are the primary source of amyloid β-peptide in human blood. *Biochem Biophys Res Commun.* **213**: 96–103.

107 Rosenberg RN, Baskin F, Fosmire JA *et al.* (1997) Altered amyloid protein processing in platelets of patients with Alzheimer disease. *Arch Neurol.* **54**: 139–44.

108 Matsubara E, Frangione B and Ghiso J (1995) Characterization of apolipoprotein J – Alzheimer's Aβ interaction. *J Biol Chem.* **270**: 7563–7.

109 Zlokovic BV (1996) Cerebrovascular transport of Alzheimer's amyloid β and apolipoproteins J and E: possible anti-amyloidogenic role of the blood–brain barrier. *Life Sci.* **59**: 1483–97.

110 Wisniewski KE, Dalton AL, Crapper McLachlan DR *et al.* (1985) Alzheimer's disease in Down's syndrome. *Neurology.* **35**: 957–61.

111 Wisniewski HM, Wegiel J and Popovitch ER (1994) Age-associated development of diffuse and thioflavin-S-positive plaques in Down syndrome. *Dev Brain Dysfunct.* **7**: 330–9.

112 Teller JK, Russo C, DeBusk LM *et al.* (1996) Presence of soluble amyloid β-peptide precedes amyloid plaque formation in Down's syndrome. *Nat Med.* **2**: 93–5.

113 Cavini S, Tamaoka A, Moretti A *et al.* (2000) Plasma levels of amyloid β 40 and 42 are independent from ApoE genotype and mental retardation in Down syndrome. *Am J Med Genet.* **95**: 224–8.

114 Tokuda T, Fukushima T, Ikeda S *et al.* (1997) Plasma levels of amyloid β proteins Aβ1–40 and Aβ1–42(43) are elevated in Down syndrome. *Ann Neurol.* **41**: 271–3.

115 Potempska A, Mack K, Mehta P *et al.* (1999) Quantification of sub-femtomole amounts of Alzheimer amyloid β peptides. *Int J Exp Clin Invest.* **16**: 14–21.

116 Gyure KA, Durham R, Stewart WF *et al.* (2001) Intraneuronal Aβ-amyloid precedes development of amyloid plaques in Down syndrome. *Arch Pathol Lab Med.* **125**: 489–92.

117 Mori C, Spooner KE, Wisniewski TM *et al.* (2002) Intraneuronal Aβ42 accumulation in Down syndrome brain. *Amyloid.* **9**: 88–102.

118 Weller RO, Massey A, Newman TA *et al.* (1998) Cerebral amyloid angiopathy: amyloid beta accumulates in putative interstitial fluid drainage pathways in Alzheimer's disease. *Am J Pathol.* **153**: 725–33.

119 Schupf N, Patel B, Silverman W *et al.* (2001) Elevated plasma amyloid β-peptide 1–42 and onset of dementia in adults with Down syndrome. *Neurosci Lett.* **301**: 199–203.

120 Harrington CR, Muketova-Ladinska EB, Hills R *et al.* (1991) Measurement of distinct immunochemical presentations of tau protein in Alzheimer's disease. *Proc Natl Acad Sci USA.* **88**: 5842–6.

121 Hof PR, Bouras C, Perl DP *et al.* (1995) Age-related distribution of neuropathologic changes in the cerebral cortex of patients with Down's syndrome. *Arch Neurol.* **52**: 379–91.

122 Hyman BT, West HL, Rebeck WG *et al.* (1995) Neuropathological changes in Down's syndrome hippocampal formation. *Arch Neurol.* **52**: 373–8.

123 Weigel J, Wisniewski HM, Dziewiatkowski J *et al.* (1996) Differential susceptibility to neurofibrillary pathology among patients with Down syndrome. *Dementia.* **7**: 135–41.

124 Growdon JH (2001) Incorporating biomarkers into clinical drug trials in Alzheimer disease. *J Alz Dis.* **3**: 287–92.

125 Black SE (1999) The search for diagnostic and progression markers in AD: so near and still too far? *Neurology.* **52**: 1533–4.

Chapter 5

Down syndrome, dementia and superoxide dismutase

Iqbal Singh and Mark J Dickinson

Introduction

Down syndrome (DS) is caused by an additional copy of chromosome 21, and it is presumably overexpression of genes coded for on this chromosome which results in the familiar phenotype that is observed, in addition to some of the well-recognised associations, including dementia in Alzheimer's disease (DAD). It represents the only trisomy compatible with long-term survival, which may be related to the relatively small size of chromosome 21 (a smaller number of enzymes and proteins are coded for and therefore fewer will be overexpressed). An additional copy of a gene is not invariably associated with overexpression of an enzyme or protein,[1] although this does seem to be the case for some, including superoxide dismutase.[2–4] In this chapter we shall examine how overexpression of superoxide dismutase may be linked to some of the problems faced by people with DS, and we shall also consider possible treatment strategies.

Superoxide dismutase

Free radicals are chemical species that have a single unpaired electron in an outer orbit. Energy created by this unstable configuration is released through reactions with adjacent molecules (proteins, lipids, carbohydrates and nucleic acids), causing damage to these molecules. Free radicals can occur as an undesirable consequence of normal respiration, or may be produced in neutrophils when activated to kill micro-organisms.

Free radicals can cause lipoperoxidation of cell membranes (damage to fats), degradation of critical enzymes within the cells (damage to proteins) and damage to DNA (possibly linked to ageing and malignant transformation of cells). The free radical, superoxide O_2^-, may be formed during the normal cellular handling of oxygen, and is itself toxic. It is converted to hydrogen peroxide (H_2O_2) by superoxide dismutase. Hydrogen peroxide is then detoxified by the enzymes catalase and glutathione peroxidase, but under conditions where this does not happen quickly enough, and in the presence of certain metals (of which iron is probably the most important), the more toxic hydroxyl OH^- radical may be produced.

The majority of the energy-yielding oxidative processes in the cell are confined to mitochondria, where the concentrations of free iron and copper are controlled by binding to storage and transport proteins (transferrin, ferritin and caerulo-plasmin), thereby minimising hydroxyl radical formation.[5,6]

In summary, superoxide dismutase together with glutathione peroxidase and catalase are the most important enzymes involved in antioxidant defence.[7,8] Such mechanisms are essential because aerobic metabolism produces highly reactive free radical molecules which cause widespread indiscriminate oxidation and peroxidation of protein, DNA and lipids.[9] They will cause cell damage and organ failure unless they are metabolised by the above-mentioned enzymes.[10]

As mentioned above, superoxide dismutase converts the superoxide radical O_2^- to hydrogen peroxide, which may then form the particularly toxic hydroxyl radical OH^- in the presence of metal ions via the Fenton reaction:[10,11]

$$O_2^- + O_2^- + 2H^+ \rightarrow H_2O_2 + O_2$$
$$Fe^{2+} + H_2O_2 \rightarrow Fe^{3+} + OH^- + OH^-.$$

Both catalase and glutathione peroxidase prevent hydroxyl radical formation by converting the hydrogen peroxide into water. It is possible that if superoxide dismutase is overactive there may be an imbalance in the above reactions, with an excess of hydrogen peroxide produced. This may then, in the presence of metal ions, result in an overproduction of hydroxyl radicals, causing serious damage to essential molecules, proteins, DNA and lipids.

As already mentioned, superoxide dismutase is overexpressed in individuals with DS. What evidence is there that this causes problems? Kedziora and colleagues[12] have reported that the level of lipid peroxides (produced by free radicals attacking fatty acids) is significantly increased in plasma from individuals with DS. Increased rates of lipoperoxidation have also been reported in the brains of people with DS[6,13] and thiobarbituric reaction products (levels of which are raised when lipoperoxidation is taking place) are present in higher concentrations in the erythrocytes of people with DS compared with normal controls.[14] Jovanovic and colleagues[15] demonstrated significantly elevated urine levels of 8-hydroxy-2-deoxyguanosine (a marker for oxidative damage to DNA) and urine levels of malondialdehyde (a marker for lipid peroxidation) in individuals with DS compared with their sibling controls. Blood samples of children with DS have been compared with those of normal controls, looking at the total load of reactive oxygen species, and the DS group was found to have significantly raised levels of reactive oxygen species.[16]

In more general terms, ageing itself may be associated with free radical activity. It seems reasonable that if there is excessive damage to proteins, DNA and lipids, all of which are fundamental biological molecules, there will be undesirable consequences. It is possible that this process takes place in people with DS at an accelerated rate due to overactivity of superoxide dismutase, and that it may be responsible for some of the characteristics of this syndrome, including premature ageing, cataract formation, and possibly the well-recognised association with presenile dementia.

Is there any evidence that raised superoxide dismutase activity and increased oxidative damage are linked? De Haan and colleagues[17] have suggested such an association, whereby excess superoxide dismutase activity relative to activity of glutathione peroxidase (which detoxifies hydrogen peroxide) may lead to the formation of hydrogen peroxide and hydroxyl radicals (OH^-), which are even more toxic (biologically) than superoxide radicals (O_2^-).

De Haan and colleagues demonstrated that superoxide dismutase 1 transfected cell lines that had elevated superoxide dismutase 1 activity compared with glutathione peroxidase 1 activity produce higher levels of hydrogen peroxide and exhibit well-characterised markers of cellular senescence (slower proliferation and altered morphology). The same authors described a significant increase in lipoperoxidation in DS fetal cells exposed to iron sulphate ($FeSO_4$) and ascorbic acid, as might be expected in conditions where excess hydrogen peroxide is produced. Iron promotes the formation of hydroxyl radicals from hydrogen peroxide, and vitamin C may shift oxidative stress towards the production of hydrogen peroxide and hydroxyl radicals.[10]

Brugge and colleagues[18] found increased activity of superoxide dismutase in the erythrocytes of individuals with DS, and a variable 'compensatory' elevation in glutathione peroxidase activity in these cells. In their study, glutathione peroxidase levels correlated with memory function, higher levels being associated with better performance.

Other authors have also reported evidence of improved cerebral performance with increased glutathione peroxidase levels. Sinet and colleagues[19] suggested a correlation between glutathione peroxidase levels and intelligence quotient (IQ) in children with DS. This evidence suggests the possible importance of glutathione peroxidase. High levels appear to be desirable, possibly related to the consequences of increased superoxide dismutase activity and excess production of hydrogen peroxide and hydroxyl radicals. Increased activity of glutathione peroxidase modifies this effect.

Superoxide dismutase and dementia in Down syndrome

It has been recognised for many years that adults with DS have an increased prevalence of presenile dementia.[20] Pathological changes similar to those of Alzheimer's disease (AD) (senile plaques, neurofibrillary tangles and cell loss) are seen in almost all people with DS over the age of 35 years, and a proportion of these individuals are subsequently diagnosed with dementia (8% aged 35–49 years, 55% aged 50–59 years and 75% aged 60 years or over).[21]

Assuming that there is a problem with the handling of free radicals in individuals with DS, why might this be associated with presenile dementia? First, there is the general principle mentioned above, that an increased rate of damage to biological molecules might be involved in the ageing process. If such accelerated damage is present throughout life, as may be the case for individuals with DS, dementing processes associated with age may appear earlier than in a normal population[22] (the brain may be particularly sensitive to this process due to the extended lifespan of its cells).

More specifically, the rate of production of amyloid β-peptide (Aβ) from amyloid precursor protein (APP) may be increased in the presence of oxidative damage,[23,24] where membrane damage secondary to lipoperoxidation allows abnormal cleavage of this protein. Thus there may be increased production of Aβ, which then forms the plaques that are seen in AD. Tabner and colleagues[25] have suggested that the degeneration and loss of nerve cells in the brain in both AD and Parkinson's disease could be due to the direct production of hydrogen peroxide during extracellular or intracellular protein aggregation (i.e. formation of Aβ and other proteins), this process possibly being augmented by raised levels of hydrogen peroxide in individuals with DS.

Busciglio and Yanker[26] have shown that in fetuses with DS, neurons generate increased levels of reactive oxygen species, leading to neuronal apoptosis, and they have suggested the possibility that a neuronal oxidative defect may predispose individuals with DS to early onset of DAD (they also showed that the death of DS neurons *in vitro* was inhibited by free radical scavengers). Other researchers have also suggested that the deposition of aggregating Aβ may trigger the neurodegenerative cascades of AD, and that free oxygen radicals are critically involved in beta-amyloidosis.[27]

Finally, although there are few well-recognised environmental risk factors for AD, head injury does appear to be important. In this instance the availability of iron may be increased (the source being blood from local intracerebral bruising), thereby increasing the rate of hydroxyl radical production, which may then lead to significant local tissue injury and dementia.[22,23]

Epilepsy, nutrition and mean red cell volume

Although the dementia in DS is described as Alzheimer-like, it has certain features that are not typical of DAD. Two particularly important ones are the development of seizures (often myoclonic but sometimes grand mal[28]), and serious swallowing difficulties associated with weight loss and inhalation pneumonia. Starvation related to the above is an important differential diagnosis, along with depression and hypothyroidism, when considering the diagnosis in a person with DS and apparent dementia. Seizures in adults with DS who have dementia occur very commonly (in approximately 80% of cases), whereas the prevalence rate for adults in the general population with DAD is approximately 10%.[29]

It is not known whether either of these problems is caused by free radical damage (to the brain or other tissues), although Willmore[30] has suggested that head injury and bruising may, through the accumulation of extravascular iron and the formation of hydroxyl radicals, be important in the genesis of post-traumatic epilepsy. It has also been shown that the intracortical injection of iron chloride ($FeCl_3$) into rats induces epileptic seizures associated with an increase in brain lipoperoxidation.[31] It is therefore possible that processes including increased free radical stress and hydroxyl radical production may explain the epilepsy found in dementia associated with DS.

It is well documented that the mean red cell corpuscular volume is raised in individuals with DS, and that this is not related to vitamin B_{12} or folate deficiency. A possible association between DAD and raised mean red cell volume has been reported.[32] Cellular swelling has been described as the first manifestation of almost all forms of cell injury, and it occurs when cells are incapable of maintaining ionic and fluid homeostasis.[5] It has been suggested that this raised mean red cell corpuscular volume could be caused by free radical stress, possibly through lipoperoxidation of membrane components altering membrane function (e.g. osmotic resistance).[33,34] It is also possible that ongoing excessive free radical stress in DS may shift the pathway of glucose utilisation of red cells from energy production to reducing power (in order to reduce oxidised glutathione, which is used to 'mop up' excess hydrogen peroxide), possibly compromising cellular ion pumps.[23,35] Although a correlation does not appear to be inevitable, it does seem that the raised mean red cell corpuscular volume seen in DS may be worth testing for when considering a diagnosis of dementia in this population[34] (for further details on the association between mean corpuscular volume and DS, *see* Chapter 6).

Therapeutic possibilities

It follows from the above that if there is a way to modify free radical activity and damage in individuals with DS, this might be protective against the development of dementia. In this respect vitamin E, a fat-soluble antioxidant, could be a good candidate. It is relatively safe, cheap and probably preferable to vitamin C (which aids the detoxification of superoxide radicals, but may shift the balance towards the production of hydrogen peroxide which, as suggested above, may already be occurring in individuals with DS[23]). Vitamin E acts as an antioxidant and free radical scavenger,[36,37] and interrupts the chain reaction of peroxidation.[8]

Dietary therapeutic interventions have been attempted in individuals with DS in the past with limited success.[37] We suggest that the reason for this may be the choice of vitamins and minerals, which included vitamin C and iron, both of which are possibly toxic in DS under normal conditions (although, of course, iron might be a very suitable treatment for anaemia). A large international multi-centre trial is currently looking at the effect of vitamin E (1000 international units twice daily for three years) in adults with DS over the age of 50 years.[38] It is well designed, double-blind, placebo controlled, and involves a relatively large number of individuals (expected sample of 400 people). The results from this study should be very helpful in assessment of the significance of free radical handling and related problems in individuals with DS.

Since, as has already been mentioned, certain functions of white cells may be mediated through the generation of free radicals at target sites (e.g. bacteria[5,6]), some caution should be exercised with regard to the use of long-term high-dose free radical scavengers. However, as with most therapeutic interventions, a balance between possible benefits and risks needs to be considered. The devastating effects of dementia on a sufferer from this disease would certainly seem to make vitamin treatments, particularly in older age groups, worth considering.

Conclusion

Adults with DS are susceptible to dementia. This is Alzheimer-like, although it has certain specific characteristics, including an association with the development of epilepsy and swallowing problems. The dementia is presumably driven by the additional genes present on chromosome 21. One such overexpressed gene is superoxide dismutase which, through a process of altered free radical stress (the production of excessive hydrogen peroxide and hydroxyl radicals specifically), may cause, or at least be involved in, the processes of accelerated ageing, cataract formation and early dementia.

The dementia may be secondary to direct damage to cellular constituents (including membranes and DNA) by hydroxyl radicals, or it may be related to abnormal metabolism of amyloid precursor protein, or a combination of both. Dementia and epilepsy tend to occur simultaneously in DS, and could be related to excess hydroxyl radical activity. The mean corpuscular volume is raised in individuals with DS, and it tends to be raised further in adults with DS with dementia. This effect could be secondary to excess hydroxyl radical activity. Free radical scavengers are readily available, safe and cheap. To date, dietary manipulations have not been successful in DS. Vitamin E might be helpful in efforts to prevent the effects of accelerated ageing and the onset of presenile dementia in this syndrome.

Clearly there are many other gene sites on chromosome 21. In this chapter we have concentrated specifically on superoxide dismutase. However, it is accepted that this is very unlikely to represent the whole picture, and other consequences of trisomy 21 will also be involved in the dementing process that is seen in the DS population.

References

1 Fairbanks D and Anderson R (1999) *Regulation of Gene Expression. Genetics, the continuity of life.* Brooks/Cole Publishing Company, Belmont, CA.
2 Brooksbank B and Balazs R (1984) Superoxide dismutase, glutathione peroxidase and lipoperoxidation in Down's syndrome fetal brain. *Dev Brain Res.* **16**: 37–44.
3 Deary I and Whalley L (1988) Recent research on the causes of Alzheimer's disease. *BMJ.* **297**: 807–10.
4 De La Torre R, Casado A, Lopez Fernandez E *et al.* (1996) Overexpression of copper–zinc superoxide dismutase in trisomy 21. *Experientia.* **52**: 871–3.
5 Cotran R, Kumar V and Collins T (1999) *Pathological Basis of Disease* (6e). WB Saunders Company, Philadelphia.
6 Stipanuk M (2001) *Biochemical and Physiological Aspects of Human Nutrition.* WB Saunders Company, Philadelphia.
7 Das D and Essman W (1990) *Oxygen Radicals: systematic events and disease processes.* Karger Press, Basel.
8 Pigeolet E, Corbisier P and Houbion A (1990) Glutathione peroxidase, superoxide dismutase, and catalase inactivation by peroxides and oxygen-derived free radicals. *Mech Age Dev.* **51**: 283–97.
9 Lehninger A (1975) *Biochemistry* (2e). Worth Publishers, Inc., London.
10 Sinclair A, Barnett A and Lunec J (1990) Free radicals and antioxidant systems in health and disease. *Br J Hosp Med.* **43**: 334–44.
11 Halliwell B and Gutteridge J (1986) Oxygen-free radicals and iron in relation to biology and medicine: some problems and concepts. *Arch Biochem Biophys.* **246**: 501–14.
12 Kedziora J, Bartosz G, Gromadzinska J *et al.* (1986) Lipid peroxides in blood and plasma and enzymatic antioxidant defence of erythrocytes in Down's syndrome. *Clin Chim Acta.* **154**: 191–4.
13 Balazs R and Brooksbank B (1985) Neurochemical approaches to the pathogenesis of Down's syndrome. *J Ment Defic Res.* **29**: 1–14.
14 Bras A, Monteiro C and Rueff J (1989) Oxidative stress in trisomy 21. A possible role in cataractogenesis. *Ophthalmic Genet.* **10**: 271–7.
15 Jovanovic S, Clements D and MacLeod K (1998) Biomarkers of oxidative stress are significantly elevated in Down syndrome. *Free Radic Biol Med.* **25**: 1044–8.
16 Carratelli M, Porcaro L, Ruscica M *et al.* (2001) Reactive oxygen metabolites and pro-oxidant status in children with Down's syndrome. *Int J Clin Pharmacol Res.* **21**: 79–84.

17 De Haan B, Cristiano F, Iannello R *et al.* (1996) Elevation in the ratio of Cu/Zn-superoxide dismutase to glutathione peroxidase activity induces features of cellular senescence and this effect is mediated by hydrogen peroxide. *Hum Mol Genet.* **5:** 283–92.

18 Brugge K, Nichols S, Saitoh T *et al.* (1999) Correlations of glutathione peroxidase activity with memory impairment in adults with Down syndrome. *Biol Psychiatry.* **46:** 1682–9.

19 Sinet P, Lejeune J and Jerome H (1979) Trisomy 21 (Down's syndrome) glutathione peroxidase, hexose monophosphate shunt and IQ. *Life Sci.* **24:** 29–34.

20 Oliver C and Holland A (1986) Down's syndrome and Alzheimer's disease: a review. *Psychol Med.* **16:** 307–22.

21 Lai F and Williams R (1989) A prospective study of Alzheimer's disease in Down's syndrome. *Arch Neurol.* **46:** 849–53.

22 Volicer L and Crino P (1990) Involvement of free radicals in dementia of the Alzheimer type: a hypothesis. *Neurobiol Aging.* **11:** 567–71.

23 Dickinson M and Singh I (1993) Down's syndrome, dementia, and superoxide dismutase. *Br J Psychiatry.* **162:** 811–17.

24 Lott I and Head E (2001) Down syndrome and Alzheimer's disease: a link between development and aging. *Ment Retard Dev Disabil Res Rev.* **7:** 172–8.

25 Tabner B, Turnbull S, El-Agnaf A *et al.* (2002) Formation of hydrogen peroxide and hydroxyl radicals from A(beta) and alpha-synuclein as a possible mechanism of cell death in Alzheimer's disease and Parkinson's disease. *Free Radic Biol Med.* **32:** 1076–83.

26 Busciglio J and Yanker B (1995) Apoptosis and increased generation of reactive oxygen species in Down's syndrome neurons *in vitro*. *Nature.* **378:** 776–9.

27 Friedlich A and Butcher L (1994) Involvement of free oxygen radicals in beta amyloidosis: a hypothesis. *Neurobiol Aging.* **15:** 443–55.

28 Vignatelli L, Meletti S and Ambrosetto G (1999) 'Progressive myoclonus epilepsy' in a Down syndrome patient with Alzheimer's disease. *Boll Lega Ital Epilessia.* **106/107:** 215–16.

29 Puri B and Singh I (2001) Age of seizure onset in adults with Down's syndrome. *Int J Clin Pract.* **55:** 442–4.

30 Willmore L (1990) Post-traumatic epilepsy: cellular mechanisms and implications for treatment. *Epilepsia.* **31 (Suppl. 3):** 67–73.

31 Singh R and Pathak D (1990) Lipid peroxidation and glutathione peroxidase, glutathione reductase, superoxide dismutase and glucose-6-phosphate dehydrogenase activities in $FeCl_3$-induced epileptogenic foci in the rat brain. *Epilepsia.* **31:** 15–26.

32 Jain S, Ross J and Levy G (1986) The accumulation of malonyldialdehyde, an end product of membrane lipid peroxidation, can cause a potassium leak in normal and sickle red blood cells. *Biochem Med Meta Biol.* **42:** 60–5.

33 Petukhov E, Filimonov M and Aleksandrova N (1990) Lipid peroxidation and disorders of erythrocyte properties in patients with mechanical jaundice. *Khirurgiia (Mosk).* **1:** 27–30.

34 Prasher V and Cheung Chung M (1993) Down's syndrome, dementia, and superoxide dismutase. *Br J Psychiatry.* **163:** 552.

35 Bindoli A, Valente M and Cavallini L (1985) Inhibition of lipid peroxidation by alpha-tocopherolquinone and alpha-tocopherolhydroquinone. *Biochem Int.* **10:** 753–61.

36 McCay P (1985) Vitamin E: interactions with free radicals and ascorbate. *Annu Rev Nutr.* **5:** 323–40.

37 Salman M (2002) Systematic review of the effect of therapeutic dietary supplements and drugs on cognitive function in subjects with Down syndrome. *Eur J Paediatr Neurol.* **6:** 213–19.

38 Aisen PS, Dalton AJ, Sano M *et al.* (2005) Design and implementation of a multicenter trial of vitamin E in aging individuals with Down syndrome. *J Policy Pract Intellect Disabil.* **2:** 86–93.

Chapter 6

Macrocytosis: a peripheral marker for dementia in Alzheimer's disease in adults with Down syndrome?

Vee P Prasher

Introduction

During the last two decades there have been a number of significant advances in our understanding and management of dementia in Alzheimer's disease (DAD), particularly in the areas of molecular genetics and drug treatment. However, the discovery of a definite genetic or clinical marker associated with Alzheimer's disease (AD) would be a huge development in the research and clinical management of this form of neurodegenerative disorder. The accurate clinical detection of early DAD in adults with Down syndrome (DS) is problematic, and the validity of diagnosis has not been researched. For the general population the identification of DAD by clinical diagnosis alone can lead to a misdiagnosis in up to 30% of cases.[1] A specific biological measure for DAD would improve the clinical diagnostic accuracy, aid early detection, improve the quality of treatment trials, increase our knowledge of the pathogenesis of the disorder and determine whether AD is a specific brain disease or a generalised system disorder. The clinical diagnosis of DAD is currently made by exclusion of other causes of dementia and intellectual decline. A biological measure would ensure that there is a 'positive' indicator of AD. A number of biological measures have been investigated, but no such measure has been established. Ideally such a measure should allow a test to be developed that uses body material which is easily accessible (e.g. urine, blood, saliva), readily discriminates DAD from other forms of intellectual decline (e.g. depressive pseudodementia, age-associated cognitive decline), has good sensitivity and specificity for DAD and is cost-effective.

However, a number of difficulties are encountered when investigating biological measures possibly associated with AD. Such difficulties are often magnified when applied to the population with intellectual disability (ID).

1   As the neuropathological findings of AD are seen in normal ageing it is highly unlikely that one single qualitative measure specific for AD will be found. It is not a matter of 'having' or 'not having' AD and a single measure being able to differentiate between the two groups. AD is a continuum disorder, and a combination of qualitative measures and quantitative scaling of a given measure may be necessary.

2 The clinical diagnosis of DAD must be as reliable as possible, as inaccurate diagnosis may lead to potential measures being missed. The diagnostic criteria must be rigid and as narrow as possible. It is possible to exclude people with possible DAD in order to ensure that the study sample has *definite* cases.

3 The severity of DAD may need to be controlled for. Although not applicable to genetic markers, it is reasonable to assume that the levels of any proposed biochemical measure are likely to be affected by the severity and duration of the disease process. It is probable that the greater the severity the greater the change in measured value will be.

4 Studies are often of a cross-sectional design. For biochemical measures, differences may be due to inter-subject variability. Norms for many measures that are investigated are not available. Longitudinal assessments and measures are necessary to show a consistent association affect.

5 Several compounding factors may need to be controlled for, such as age, gender, underlying level of intelligence, coincidental illness, phase of illness and medication.

6 Tests must be relatively simple to undertake, cost-effective, reliable, specific and non-traumatic. They should not require hospitalisation and should be widely available.

Several blood biological measures associated with DAD in the general population have been proposed (*see* Table 6.1). Any given association is more robust if the measure has been positively associated in several studies. However, in the case of biochemical measures a positive association has often been demonstrated only in single studies and has not been confirmed by other researchers.

It is not unreasonable to assume that for any given biochemical measure to be a valid marker of DAD, there must be a rational link between a disease affecting the brain and the associated measure. This particularly applies to biochemical changes observed outside the central nervous system where, although AD is localised to the brain, it must be directly or indirectly linked to changes seen in the periphery. To this end, a number of researchers have argued that DAD is one aspect of a multi-functional systemic disorder rather than a localised disease entity in its own right.[31] The characteristic neuropathological changes seen in AD may represent an end-stage immune reaction resulting from a systemic disorder.

If, as is generally accepted, AD in adults with DS is the same disease process as that seen in the general population, it would seem reasonable to assume that any identified genetic or biochemical measure should show some degree of abnormality in both populations. For many reasons, comparable research into biological measures associated with DAD in the general population has not been undertaken in the ID population. For example, ethical committee approval and the obtaining of informed consent for a research study of DAD in individuals with DS is problematic. The available population of DS adults with DAD for research is relatively small compared with the number of individuals with DAD available in the general population. Accurate and early diagnosis of DAD in adults with DS remains difficult.

The most researched body material is blood, and some of the blood measures investigated in the general population are already known to be abnormal in the DS population. As such these measures may prove to be possible markers for AD in the two populations. One blood measure that has shown to be a potential

Table 6.1 Possible peripheral measures for Alzheimer's disease

Measure	Finding
Endocrine	
Dexamethasone suppression test	Impaired[2]
Calcium homeostasis	Impaired[3,4]
Growth hormone secretion	Altered[5]
Thyroid function	Impaired[6]
Plasma/serum	
Inorganic sulphate concentration	Reduced[7]
Immunoglobulins (IgA, IgG)	Elevated[8–10]
Alpha-1-antichymotrypsin	Elevated[11,12]
Interleukin-1 production	Reduced[13]
Amyloid A protein	Elevated[14]
Albumin/prealbumin	Reduced[14]
Vitamin B_{12}	Reduced[15]
Protein p97	Increased[16]
Red blood cells	
Acetylcholine	Elevated[17,18]
Choline acetyltransferase	Elevated[17]
Superoxide dismutase activity	Elevated[19]
Glutathione peroxidase activity	Elevated[20,21]
Red blood cell/plasma choline ratio	Elevated[17,22]
Size and shape	Increased distortion
White blood cells	
Total lymphocyte count	Reduced[23]
Lymphocytic action	Impaired[24–26]
Platelets	
Membrane fluidity	Increased[27,28]
Number	Increased[29]
Serotonin metabolism	Altered[29]
Enzyme action	Altered[30]

biological marker for DAD in adults with DS is change in red blood cell size and shape. The significance of these abnormalities will be reviewed in this chapter.

Red blood cell changes: macrocytosis

A limited number of research publications have investigated an association between DAD and red blood cell abnormalities. Goodall and colleagues[32,33] were the first research group to report on changes in red cell morphology as a measure for DAD, when they observed abnormally shaped red blood cells in adults with DAD in the general population. They examined the red blood cells in 50 patients with DAD (age range, 58–95 years; mean age of demented subjects, 81.0 years) together with cells from 100 age- and gender-matched controls from the general population.

A statistically significant (at 5% level) proportion of the demented group (14%) had abnormalities in the shape of red blood cell compared with controls (5%). The authors also highlighted the fact that red blood cell abnormalities were seen in one case several years before a diagnosis of DAD was made. The authors did not investigate the cause of the red cell abnormalities further, but suggested that these abnormalities were secondary to cell membrane dysfunction. These findings for individuals with DAD in the general population have not been confirmed by subsequent research.

Several years before the findings for the general population were reported by Goodall and colleagues,[32,33] abnormalities in the morphology of red blood cells had been reported to occur in individuals with DS. An increase in mean corpuscular volume (MCV) compared with the general population was the principal finding. Eastham and Jancar[34,35] reported the presence of macrocytosis (mean MCV 102.5 ± 7.87fl) in 92 adults with DS who were prescribed anticonvulsant medication, and later the same authors reported macrocytosis in 33 adults with DS who were not on anticonvulsant medication (mean MCV 96.3 ± 3.79 fl). These values were above the accepted upper limit of the normal range for their laboratory (95 fl). The authors did not go on to investigate the possible cause of an association between DS and macrocytosis, but did comment that it may be due to accelerated ageing.

Support for an association between DS and macrocytosis was provided by Hewitt and colleagues[36] when they confirmed the finding by Eastham and Jancar[34,35] of an association between macrocytosis and DS. Hewitt and colleagues[36] recruited 23 hospital patients with DS aged 50 years or over. Not only was the average MCV for the group above that for the general population (mean, 95.4 fl; upper limit, 96 fl), but for 11 individuals their MCV result was above the upper limit of the range for the general population. The authors also investigated the hypothesis proposed by Eastham and Jancar[35] that macrocytosis is a measure of accelerated ageing. The mental age of the subjects was assessed on several occasions using the Stanford Binet Intelligence Scale.[37] Repeat assessments allowed deterioration in mental function to be monitored. For nine of the patients who showed evidence of intellectual deterioration, their MCV measurement was higher than the mean MCV for the sample as a whole. Only two patients with no evidence of mental deterioration had raised MCV values. Eastham and Jancar[34,35] therefore found a significant association between intellectual decline and macrocytosis, but as they did not assess the presence of DAD, no link between macrocytosis and DAD could be made.

Lansdall-Welfare and Hewitt[38] later investigated an association between macrocytosis and DS in 23 patients living in an institution for people with ID. The authors found that the mean MCV for individuals with intellectual deterioration was 100.23 fl (range 92–106 fl), compared with 95.14 fl (range 91–103.2 fl) for those without intellectual deterioration. This difference was statistically significant ($P <$ 0.005). However, Hewitt and colleagues did not assess for the presence or absence of dementia, so again a direct link between macrocytosis and DAD could not be made.

Although the above studies were of limited methodological validity, there was now growing evidence in support of an association between macrocytosis and DS, and in particular between macrocytosis and intellectual deterioration in adults with DS. The reported studies to date had not differentiated between individuals with and without DAD when investigating a link between macrocytosis and intellectual decline. As a result, it was impossible to determine whether macrocytosis was associated with DAD in older adults with DS or was a measure for ageing per se. Prasher[39-41] in a number of studies specifically investigated the possibility of the former association.

Prasher[39] initially reported findings from an investigation of a large cross-sectional study. MCV measurements were available for 147 individuals out of a sample of 201 adults who were assessed for DAD using *ICD–10* criteria.[42] A total of 27 individuals were diagnosed with DAD (mean age, 54.1 years; age range, 39–72 years). The mean MCV value for the 147 subjects was 99.28 fl (SD, 5.80; SE, 0.48; range, 77.5–116 fl), the upper limit of the normal range being 98.0 fl. In total, 70 individuals had MCV values above this upper limit (> 98.0 fl). There was no statistically significant correlation between MCV and age (Pearson's product–moment coefficient = 0.041; $P = 0.62$). A total of 66 subjects were found to have neither DAD nor macrocytosis, 54 individuals did not have DAD but did have macrocytosis, 10 subjects had DAD but did not have macrocytosis, and 17 individuals had DAD and macrocytosis. A borderline statistically significant association was found between macrocytosis and DAD (Chi-square test; $P = 0.05$). Prasher[39] proposed that macrocytosis in adults with DS was associated with DAD and could possibly be a peripheral measure for DAD.

In a later study, Prasher[40] went on to investigate changes in MCV over time in adults with DS with and without DAD. A total of 17 adults (all trisomy 21) with a diagnosis of DAD according to *ICD–10* criteria[42] were matched for age and gender with 17 non-demented DS controls. The mean age of the DAD group was 55.5 years (SD = 8.2 years) at the start of the study. In total, 12 individuals had mild DAD, two had moderate DAD and three had severe DAD at the start of the study, but after one year only five individuals had mild dementia, nine had moderate DAD and three had severe DAD. The mean duration of DAD at the start was 1.4 years. The MCV was measured at a given time point and again one year later for all subjects.

The mean MCV at the start was 97.5 fl for the DAD group and 94.3 fl for the control group (borderline statistical significance; $P = 0.54$). One year later the mean MCV for the DAD group was 98.7 fl and that for the control group was 94.5 fl (statistically significant; $P = 0.03$). The findings suggested that as the severity and duration of DAD increased so did the MCV. Therefore macrocytosis could be a potential marker for change in DAD.

Prasher and colleagues[41] went on to investigate further an association between DAD in adults with DS and macrocytosis, and correlated longitudinal changes in MCV levels with deterioration in DAD over a 5-year study period. A total of 150 adults with DS participated in this study, of whom 83 (55%) were male and 67 (45%) were female. The mean age of the total sample population at year 1 was 44.0 years (SD = 11.46; SE = 0.93; range, 16–76 years). For men the mean age was 42.4 years (SD = 11.22; SE = 1.23; range, 16–72 years) and for women the mean age was 50.0 years (SD = 11.55; SE = 1.41; range, 19–76 years). A total of 44 individuals were diagnosed with DAD during the 5-year study period. For 140 subjects at least one MCV result was available for analysis during the 5-year period. In total 512 data cells were available for analysis (subjects x time period). Results were available for 116 subjects at year 1, for 98 subjects at year 2, for 102 subjects at year 3, for 96 subjects at year 4 and for 100 subjects at year 5. Poor compliance with venepuncture and death of subjects during the study period were the principal reasons for missing data.

The mean MCV value for the sample for which results were available was 97.33 fl (SD = 5.27; range, 77.50–115.90 fl). This was at the upper limit of the normal range for the general population (78–99 fl). For subjects who had no significant medical disorder, an association was found between MCV and age (Pearson's correlation coefficient; $P < 0.05$), but this was accounted for by gender (i.e. if gender was included in the analysis no age effect was seen) (Pearson's correlation coefficient; $P = 0.54$).

The 512 data-cell MCV measurements were subdivided into those for subjects with no evidence of DAD during the study period (non-dementia group; $n = 388$), subjects who developed dementia during the study period (new dementia group; $n = 62$) and subjects who had dementia throughout the study period (persistent dementia group; $n = 62$). Statistical analysis to control for patient variability, for different subjects contributing to the data set in different years and for variation between dementia groups was undertaken. The non-dementia group had an adjusted mean MCV value of 96.73 fl (SD = 5.23; range, 77.5–115.9 fl). The new dementia group had an adjusted mean MCV value of 97.73 fl (SD = 4.87; range, 84.3–108.4 fl) and the persistent dementia group had an adjusted mean MCV value of 100.71 fl (SD = 4.59; range, 90.2–111.7 fl). There was a significant difference in mean MCV scores ($P = 0.002$), demonstrating an association between macrocytosis and DAD in adults with DS.

Gender was shown to have a significant effect on MCV. For non-demented men in the study a mean MCV value of 96.44 fl (SEM = 0.21) was found, and for non-demented women the corresponding value was 97.5 fl (SEM = 0.36). For men with persistent dementia the mean MCV value was 99.35 fl (SEM = 0.51), and for women with persistent dementia the corresponding value was 102.6 fl (SEM = 0.79). Both sets of results were statistically significantly different ($P < 0.001$), the MCV being greater for women than for men.

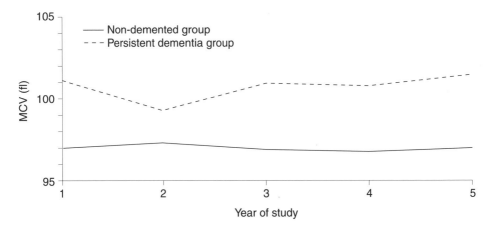

Figure 6.1 Longitudinal mean corpuscular volume findings for sample. Modified from Prasher VP, Viswanathan J and Holder R (2002) Down's syndrome, dementia and macrocytosis. *Ir J Psychol Med.* **19**: 118.

The longitudinal mean MCV values for the non-dementia group and for the persistent dementia group over the 5-year study period are shown in Figure 6.1. The values for the latter group were consistently higher.

Prasher and colleagues[41] then went on to determine cut-off points for MCV values that could separate the non-dementia group from the persistent dementia group. Sensitivity and specificity values were calculated for various cut-off points (*see* Table 6.2). Receiver operating characteristic curves were plotted (*see* Figure 6.2) in order to determine the optimum MCV value for differentiating demented from non-demented individuals with DS. The most accurate measure for DAD in men with DS would be an MCV level higher than 97 fl (sensitivity of 70% and

Table 6.2 Sensitivity and specificity for different MCV levels in men and women

MCV level (fl)	Men				Women			
	Sensitivity (%)	Specificity (%)	PPV (%)	NPV (%)	Sensitivity (%)	Specificity (%)	PPV (%)	NPV (%)
>96	76	46	20	90	97	40	27	87
>97	70	59	24	91	89	52	29	85
>98	65	67	27	91	89	57	30	85
>99	52	76	28	89	78	63	30	83
>100	46	81	31	89	68	71	33	83
>101	42	85	34	89	68	76	37	84
>102	33	90	39	88	46	78	33	81

PPV, positive predictive value; NPV, negative predictive value.
Table modified from Prasher VP, Viswanathan J and Holder R (2002) Down's syndrome, dementia and macrocytosis. *Ir J Psychol Med.* **19**: 117.

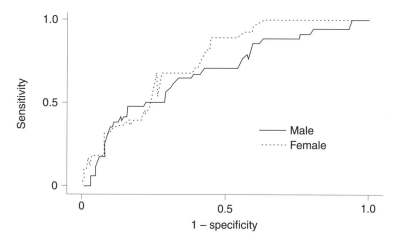

Figure 6.2 Receiver operating characteristic curves for male and female subjects. Modified from Prasher VP, Viswanathan J and Holder R (2002) Down's syndrome, dementia and macrocytosis. *Ir J Psychol Med.* **19**: 119.

specificity of 59%), and for women it would be a level higher than 99 fl (sensitivity of 78% and specificity of 60%).

Prasher and colleagues[41] concluded that there was an association between macrocytosis and DAD in adults with DS. A raised MCV could be an ante-mortem measure for DAD. However, a single MCV reading has little diagnostic validity and cannot be used on its own as an accurate test for DAD. A reading above 97 fl for men and above 99 fl for women could be used as an adjunct to the clinical assessment of AD in adults with DS, but cannot be used to replace the standard assessment. An MCV result above the upper limit of the normal range (> 99 fl) in a DS patient with suspected DAD may support the diagnosis. Prasher and colleagues suggested that for all adults with DS in whom dementia was suspected, a blood test for MCV should be undertaken and used with caution to aid the clinical diagnosis of DAD.

Burt and colleagues[43] undertook a review of the data from their longitudinal study in order to confirm or refute the findings of Prasher and colleagues[41] with regard to the association between macrocytosis and DAD, and also to investigate the cut-off levels of MCV as measures for DAD. As part of their longitudinal study on dementia, the authors collected yearly laboratory data from 44 women and 32 men with DS over a 5-year period. Therefore Burt and colleagues[43] were able to examine the proposed relationship between dementia status and a number of peripheral measures. Of all of these measures, MCV was the one most consistently related to dementia status across diagnostic methods (logistic regression; $P < 0.05$). In addition, their sensitivity values were similar to those reported by Prasher and colleagues.[41] Initially Burt and colleagues[43] examined sensitivity and specificity by using any raised yearly MCV value as an indication of risk for dementia. Using the cut-off MCV values (women, > 99 fl; men, > 97 fl) subjects were classified as demented or non-demented, and the findings were compared with the clinical diagnosis. For women the sensitivity was 78% and the specificity was 50%, whereas for men the sensitivity was 83% and the specificity was 35%. When the last MCV value collected was used as an indication of risk, the sensitivity for both women and men decreased (to 56% and 66%, respectively), whereas the specificity increased (to 71% and 46%, respectively).

Thus the findings by Burt and colleagues[43] were consistent with those found by Prasher and colleagues.[41] They support a possible association between dementia in adults with DS and macrocytosis, and suggest that measurement of MCV values may improve the clinical diagnosis of dementia in adults with DS.

Causes of macrocytosis

The specific cause of macrocytosis in adults with DS is not yet known and has not been fully investigated by researchers. The commonest cause of a raised MCV value in the general population is nutritional deficiency (vitamin B_{12} and/or folate deficiency). However, findings from studies of adults with DS suggest that macrocytosis occurs independently of anaemia, vitamin B_{12} or folate deficiency.[40,41,44,45] Prasher and colleagues[41] found no statistically significant difference in serum vitamin B_{12} levels between demented and non-demented individuals with DS (t-test: t-value = 0.1; $P > 0.05$). The mean serum vitamin B_{12} concentration was 416 ng/l (SD = 155; range, 175–878 ng/l) for non-DAD subjects and 423 ng/l (SD = 121; range, 308–623 ng/l) for DAD subjects, the normal range for serum vitamin B_{12} concentration being 160–1100 ng/l. Similarly, no statistically significant difference was found between the two groups for serum folate concentration (t-test: t-value = 0.18; $P > 0.05$). The mean serum folate level was 6.2 µg/l (SD = 3.4; range, 1.9–19.5 µg/l) for non-DAD subjects and 5.9 µg/l (SD = 3.5; range, 3.3–11.9 µg/l) for DAD subjects, the normal range for serum folate concentration being 1.5–20.0 µg/l. None of the subjects in this study were found to be vitamin B_{12} or folate deficient.

Furthermore, Wachtel and Pueschel[45] had demonstrated earlier that an important factor in adults with DS was a reduced lifespan of red blood cells. For those patients who were tested for red blood cell survival time ($n = 10$), the time was found to be shorter than that for general population controls. Although the study used only a small sample, the findings indicated that accelerated ageing of red blood cells was a factor in the development of macrocytosis.

Other causes of a raised MCV value, such as alcohol abuse, blood dyscrasias, untreated hypothyroidism, chronic hepatitis and drug-related causes (e.g. use of phenytoin) have not been found in studies to date.

Discussion

The methodological difficulties discussed previously (e.g. small sample size, validity of DAD diagnosis) apply to research investigating a possible association between macrocytosis and DAD in the DS population. However, on the basis of the limited information available from both the general population and the population with ID, macrocytosis appears to be a potential peripheral measure associated with DAD, and more so for the DS population than for the general population. There may be an as yet unidentified underlying biochemical disorder that leads both to an increase in MCV by reducing the lifespan of red cells, and to the neuropathological changes of AD. Although the underlying pathophysiology of an association between macrocytosis and DAD is not well understood, a number of hypotheses have been proposed.

1 Increased activity of superoxide dismutase-1 (SOD-1), resulting in overproduction of hydrogen peroxide and hydroxyl radicals, which disrupt cellular functioning and subsequently lead to intellectual impairment and changes in MCV, has been postulated.[46]
2 Bosman and colleagues[47] investigated red cell membrane function in 31 adults with DS, of whom 12 subjects had no signs of clinical dementia (mean age, 27 ± 4 years), 10 subjects had early signs of clinical dementia (mean age, 54 ± 6 years) and 9 subjects had advanced dementia (mean age, 62 ± 6 years). Abnormalities in erythrocyte-protein IgG and enhanced breakdown of anion membrane transporter band 3 were found in the demented subjects. The authors postulated that such findings were associated with altered red blood cell ageing leading to a reduction in the lifespan of red blood cells and higher numbers of large red blood cells in the blood.
3 Increased activity of the cellular enzymes adenosine deaminase and glucose-6-phosphate dehydrogenase, leading to red cell dysfunction and abnormalities in cell size and impairment of intellectual functioning, has been postulated.

Conclusion

To date, little interest has been shown in the possible association between macrocytosis and DAD, both in the general population and in the DS population. There is now reasonable evidence in support of an association between macrocytosis and DS and possibly DAD.[35,36,41,45] Further investigation of the association between macrocytosis and DS may further improve our understanding of AD and result in improvement in diagnosis and possibly also in treatment. The underlying physiological mechanisms leading to a possible association between a raised MCV and DAD have yet to be fully investigated. Several mechanisms have been suggested, including an increase in free radical activity, abnormalities in immunoglobulin action and enzyme dysfunction.[46–48] All of them may lead to defective DNA synthesis or accelerated erythropoiesis, resulting in an increase in red cell volume.[49]

Macrocytosis may be a sign of premature ageing, a condition previously associated with DS.[50] Okamoto and colleagues[51] have previously reported macrocytosis as part of a 'premature ageing syndrome.' It is possible that macrocytosis and DAD in adults with DS are 'symptoms' of premature ageing. The specificity and sensitivity of measurement of a single MCV value are too low for the measurement of MCV to be an accurate diagnostic test for DAD in the DS population. However, the measurement of MCV together with the clinical assessment may aid the diagnosis.

References

1 Burns A (1991) Clinical diagnosis of Alzheimer's disease. *Dementia.* **2**: 186–94.
2 Jenike MA and Albert MS (1984) The dexamethasone suppression test in patients with presenile and senile dementia of the Alzheimer's type. *J Am Geriatr Soc.* **32**: 441–4.
3 Ferrier IN, Leake A, Taylor GA *et al.* (1990) Reduced gastrointestinal absorption of calcium in dementia. *Age Ageing.* **19**: 368–75.
4 Hajimohammadreza I, Brammer MJ, Eagger S *et al.* (1990) Platelet and erythrocyte membrane changes in Alzheimer's disease. *Biochim Biophys Acta.* **1025**: 208–14.
5 Christie JE, Whalley LJ, Bennie J *et al.* (1987) Characteristic plasma hormone changes in Alzheimer's disease. *Br J Psychiatry.* **150**: 674–81.
6 Thomas DR, Hailwood R, Harris B *et al.* (1987) Thyroid status in senile dementia of the Alzheimer type (SDAT). *Acta Psychiatr Scand.* **76**: 158–63.
7 Heafield MT, Fearn S, Steventon GB *et al.* (1990). Plasma cysteine and sulphate levels in patients with motor neurone, Parkinson's and Alzheimer's disease. *Neurosci Lett.* **110**: 216–20.
8 Smith NKG and Powell RJ (1985) Immunological tests and the diagnosis of dementia in elderly women. *Age Ageing.* **14**: 91–5.
9 Ounanian A, Guilbert B, Renversez J-C *et al.* (1990) Antibodies to viral antigens, xenoantigens and autoantigens in Alzheimer's disease. *J Clin Lab Anal.* **4**: 367–75.
10 Frecker MF, Pryse-Phillips WEM and Strong HR (1994) Immunological associations in familial and non-familial Alzheimer patients and their families. *Can J Neurol Sci.* **21**: 112–19.
11 Lieberman J, Schleissner L, Tachiki KH *et al.* (1995) Serum alpha-1-antichymotrypsin level as a marker for Alzheimer-type dementia. *Neurobiol Aging.* **16**: 747–53.
12 Matsubara E, Amari M, Shoji M *et al.* (1989) Serum concentration of alpha-1-antichymotrypsin is elevated in patients with senile dementia of the Alzheimer type. In: *Alzheimer's Disease and Related Disorders.* AR Liss Inc., New York.

13 Khansari N, Whitten HD, Chou YK *et al.* (1985) Immunological dysfunction in Alzheimer's disease. *J Neuroimmunol.* **7**: 279–85.

14 Elovaara I, Maury CPJ and Palo J (1986) Serum amyloid A protein, albumin and prealbumin in Alzheimer's disease and in demented patients with Down's syndrome. *Acta Neurol Scand.* **74**: 245–50.

15 Cole MG and Prachal JF (1984) Low serum vitamin B_{12} in Alzheimer-type dementia. *Age Ageing.* **13**: 101–5.

16 Kennard ML, Feldman H, Yamada T *et al.* (1996) Serum levels of the iron-binding protein p97 are elevated in Alzheimer's disease. *Nature Med.* **2**: 1230–5.

17 Hanin I, Reynolds CF III, Kupfer DJ *et al.* (1984) Elevated red blood cell/plasma choline ratio in dementia of the Alzheimer type: clinical and polysomnographic correlates. *Psychiatry Res.* **13**: 167–73.

18 Greenwald BS, Mathe AA, Mohs RC *et al.* (1986) Alzheimer's disease, dexamethasone suppression, dementia severity and affective symptoms. *Am J Psychiatry.* **143**: 442–6.

19 Sinet PM (1982) Metabolism of oxygen derivatives in Down's syndrome. *Ann N Y Acad Sci.* **396**: 83–94.

20 Marcus DL, Thomas C, Rodriguez C *et al.* (1998) Increased peroxidation and reduced antioxidant enzyme activity in Alzheimer's disease. *Exp Neurol.* **150**: 40–4.

21 Subbarao KV, Richardson JS and Ang L (1990) Autopsy samples of Alzheimer's cortex show increased peroxidation *in vitro*. *J Neurochem.* **55**: 342–5.

22 Blass JP, Hanin I, Barclay L *et al.* (1985) Red blood cell abnormalities in Alzheimer disease. *J Am Geriatr Soc.* **33**: 401–5.

23 MacDonald SM, Goldstone AH, Morris JE *et al.* (1982) Immunological parameters in the aged and in Alzheimer's disease. *Clin Exp Immunol.* **49**: 123–8.

24 Tavolato B and Argentiero V (1980) Immunological indices in presenile Alzheimer disease. *J Neurol Sci.* **46**: 325–31.

25 Jarvik LF, Matsuyama SS, Kessler JO *et al.* (1982) Philothermal response of poly-morphonuclear leukocytes in dementia of the Alzheimer type. *Neurobiol Aging.* **3**: 93–9.

26 Cameron DJ, Durst GG and Majeski JA (1985) Macrophage and polymorphonuclear leukocyte function in patients with Alzheimer disease. *Biomed Pharmacother.* **39**: 310–14.

27 Zubenko GS, Cohen BM, Boller F *et al.* (1987) Platelet membrane abnormality in Alzheimer's disease. *Ann Neurol.* **22**: 237–44.

28 Kukull WA, Hinds TR, Schellenberg GD *et al.* (1992) Increased platelet membrane fluidity as a diagnostic marker for Alzheimer's disease: a test in population-based cases and controls. *Neurology.* **42**: 607–14.

29 Inestrosa NC, Alacron R, Arriagda J *et al.* (1993) Platelets of Alzheimer patients: increased counts and subnormal uptake and accumulation of [^{14}C]5-hydroxytrypta-mine. *Neurosci Lett.* **163**: 8–10.

30 Hollander E, Mohs E and Davis KL (1986) Antemortem markers of Alzheimer's disease. *Neurobiol Aging.* **7**: 367–87.

31 Sweet RA and Zubenko GS (1994) Peripheral markers in Alzheimer's disease. In: A Burns and R Levy (eds) *Dementia.* Chapman and Hall, London.

32 Goodall HB, McHarg JF, Anderson JM *et al.* (1991) Acanthocytosis in disparate clinical states – myelodysplasia and Alzheimer's disease. *Leuk Res.* **15 (Suppl. 2)**: 19.

33 Goodall HB, Reid AH, Findlay DJ *et al.* (1994) Irregular distortion of the erythrocytes (acanthocytes, spur cells) in senile dementia. *Dis Markers.* **12**: 23–41.

34 Eastham RD and Jancar J (1970) Macrocytosis in Down's syndrome and during long-term anticonvulsant therapy. *J Clin Pathol.* **23**: 296–8.

35 Eastham RD and Jancar J (1983) Macrocytosis and Down syndrome. *Br J Psychiatry.* **143**: 203–4.

36 Hewitt KE, Carter G and Jancer J (1985) Ageing in Down's syndrome. *Br J Psychiatry.* **147**: 58–62.

37 Terman LM and Merrill MA (1937) *Measuring Intelligence*. Houghton Mifflin, Boston, MA.

38 Lansdall-Welfare RW and Hewitt KE (1986) Macrocytosis and cognitive decline in Down's syndrome. *Br J Psychiatry*. **148:** 482–3.

39 Prasher VP (1994) Down syndrome, dementia and macrocytosis. *Br J Dev Disabil*. **90:** 131–4.

40 Prasher VP (1997) Increase in mean cell volume: a possible peripheral marker for Alzheimer's disease? *Int J Geriatr Psychiatry*. **12:** 130–1.

41 Prasher VP, Viswanathan J and Holder R (2002) Down syndrome, dementia and macrocytosis. *Ir J Psychol Med*. **19:** 115–20.

42 World Health Organization (1993) *ICD–10 Classification of Mental and Behavioural Disorders. Diagnostic criteria for research*. World Health Organization, Geneva.

43 Burt D, Loveland K, Lewis K and Lesser J (2003) Macrocytosis: a marker for Alzheimer's in adults with Down's syndrome. *Ir J Psychol Med*. **20:** 135–6.

44 Akin K (1988) Macrocytosis and leukopenia in Down's syndrome. *JAMA*. **259:** 842.

45 Wachtel TJ and Peuschel SM (1991) Macrocytosis in Down syndrome. *Am J Ment Retard*. **95:** 417–20.

46 Dickinson MJ and Singh I (1993) Down's syndrome, dementia and superoxide dismutase. *Br J Psychiatry*. **162:** 811–17.

47 Bosman GJ, Visser FE, De Man AJM *et al.* (1993) Erythrocyte membrane changes of individuals with Down's syndrome in various stages of Alzheimer-type dementia. *Neurobiol Aging*. **14:** 223–8.

48 Pastor MC, Sierra C, Dolade M *et al.* (1998) Antioxidant enzymes and fatty acid status in erythrocytes of Down's syndrome patients. *Clin Chem*. **44:** 924–9.

49 Lee GR, Bithell TC, Foerster J *et al.* (1993) *Clinical Hematology*. Lea and Febiger, Philadephia, PA.

50 Nakamura E and Tanaka S (1998) Biological ages of adult men and women with Down's syndrome and its changes with aging. *Mech Ageing Dev*. **105:** 89–103.

51 Okamoto N, Satomura K, Hatsukawa Y *et al.* (1997) Premature aging syndrome with osteosarcoma, cataracts, diabetes mellitus, osteoporosis, erythroid macrocytosis, severe growth and developmental deficiency. *Am J Med Genet*. **69:** 169–70.

Chapter 7

Thyroid disorders, dementia and Down syndrome

Maire Percy and Vee P Prasher

Introduction

A long-standing association between Down syndrome (DS) and thyroid disorders has been well documented in the literature.[1-27] However, because of uncertainty about what to use as normal reference levels for interpretation of test results on people with DS, the question of whether or not these individuals have an unusually high prevalence of thyroid dysfunction has recently been raised.[19] The relationship between dementia and thyroid dysfunction in Alzheimer's disease (AD) in the general population has for many years been the focus of considerable clinical and research interest.[28-72] Because people with DS are at risk of developing dementia in Alzheimer's disease (DAD) 20–30 years earlier than in the general population (*see* Chapter 1), the question of whether or not there is a relationship between thyroid dysfunction and DAD in DS has also been a focus of interest.[16,17,73-77] An understanding of thyroid disease in individuals with DS who are at high risk of developing DAD is essential in order to ensure the provision of optimum care for patients with dementia.

Before reviewing the possible association between thyroid disorders and AD, this chapter will discuss thyroid function in general, including the following topics:

1 the main functions of the thyroid gland[78-116]
2 tests for thyroid function[11,78,101,103-106,111,117]
3 abnormalities of thyroid function in the general population[24,29,78,81,83, 95-97,106-108,118-128] and in DS[1-3,5-9,11-13,15-19,21-27,129]
4 the controversial issue of subclinical hypothyroidism and whether or not to treat it in the general population[130-134] and in individuals with DS[8,9,15,19,26]
5 involvement of the thyroid in AD in the general population[15-17,28-37,39-53,55,73,74,75,135] and in DS[15,16,17,73,74,75]
6 strategies for managing thyroid dysfunction,[130,136-144] especially in people with DS,[9,11,19,145-147] including studies of oral supplementation with selenium and zinc in individuals with DS, and other approaches.[25,148-173]

The thyroid gland and its functions

Importance of thyroid function

Thyroid dysfunction is possibly the most important topic in endocrinology. Normal thyroid function is essential not only for normal physical growth and brain development, but also for regulation of the rate of metabolic reactions in the body throughout the lifespan, and for neural activity. Thyroid hormone effects include increasing the body's overall metabolic rate, increasing heat production, increasing target-cell responsiveness to catecholamines (adrenaline and noradrenaline) and acetylcholine, increasing the heart stroke volume and heart rate, having an effect on growth hormone action, and promoting normal myelination and development of the nervous system.[98,113]

Thyroid dysfunction may occur at any age. It should be treated in the earliest possible stages, when it is reversible.[28,29,174,175] Correcting hypothyroidism, even if mild, during pregnancy is key to normal fetal development. Fetuses do not acquire the ability to synthesise thyroid hormones until 10–12 weeks of age, but during pregnancy there is substantial transfer of maternal thyroid hormones across the placenta.[82,93,116] The next opportunity for correcting thyroid dysfunction is shortly after birth.

The thyroid gland

The thyroid gland is located at the base of the throat. It is butterfly-shaped and weighs 15–25 g, the right lobe being larger than the left. It is composed of many follicles which contain colloid surrounded by a single layer of epithelium. In addition to a person's genetic make-up, a number of other factors and processes affect function of the thyroid. These include thyroid hormone production; binding of thyroid hormone and derivatives to receptors; the availability of iodine, iron, selenium and zinc; thyroid-hormone-binding proteins; thyroid hormone degradation and the hypothalamic–pituitary–thyroid (HPT) axis.[106,107]

Thyroid hormone production

The following processes are involved in the production of thyroid hormones. Ingested iodine is absorbed through the small intestine and transported in the plasma to the thyroid. There it is concentrated, oxidised and incorporated into thyroglobulin (Tg) under the action of haem-containing thyroperoxidase, which uses hydrogen peroxide as a substrate. Iodide attaches to tyrosine residues in Tg, and iodinated tyrosine residues couple to form thyroid hormone precursor, which is stored in thyroid follicles. When hormone is needed, the hormone precursor is endocytosed by the follicular epithelial cells, hydrolysed in lysosomes and the released hormones are secreted into the circulation where specific binding proteins carry them to target tissues. Thyroxine (T4) is the precursor of triiodothyronine (T3), the most active thyroid hormone (the numbers 3 and 4 indicate the number of iodinated tyrosine residues that are present in the hormone molecules). T3 is more potent than T4, but levels of T4 are about 50-fold higher than those of T3.[102,106,107]

How thyroid hormones exert their effect

T3 exerts its effect by crossing the cell membrane and binding to a receptor in the cell nucleus. The receptors then bind to DNA at sites in the 5′ untranslated regions of thyroid-hormone-responsive genes called thyroid response elements. Interaction of T3 with its receptor causes the binding of accessory protein cofactors that either activate or repress a specific gene's transcription.[85,91,106,107,113] One example of a gene whose transcription is upregulated as a result of T3 stimulation is that for Na^+/K^+-ATPase, to increase oxidative metabolism.[176] An example of a gene whose transcription is downregulated as a result of T3 stimulation is that for amyloid precursor protein (APP).[30,72]

Non-genetic factors that affect levels and/or activity of thyroid hormones

Availability of iodine and trace elements

Thyroid function is dependent upon the availability of iodine and several other trace elements. The relationship between the iodine intake level of a population and the occurrence of thyroid diseases is U-shaped, with an increase in risk associated with both low and high iodine intake. At the low end of the spectrum, severe iodine deficiency leads to endemic goitre (swelling in the neck due to an enlarged thyroid gland), cretinism (a congenital form of thyroid hormone deficiency that retards mental and physical growth) and developmental brain disorders in young children, a spectrum of disorders sometimes referred to as fetal iodine-deficiency disorder. The features of cretinism include a puffy face, open mouth with large protruding tongue, short thick neck, narrow forehead, pug nose, short legs, distended abdomen, hoarse voice, dry yellowish skin, excessive hairiness, lethargy and intellectual disability. Less severe iodine deficiency is associated with multinodular autonomous growth and function of the thyroid gland, leading to goitre and hypothyroidism in middle-aged and elderly subjects. Extremely excessive iodine intake is associated with a high prevalence of thyroid hypofunction and goitre in children. Moderate and mild iodine excesses are associated with a more frequent occurrence of hypothyroidism, especially in elderly people. Fetal iodine-deficiency disorder is the commonest cause of intellectual disability worldwide.[95–97,177] The supplementation of salt with iodine, introduced in the 1920s, has markedly reduced the frequency of fetal iodine-deficiency disorder and thyroid disorders in older individuals resulting from iodine deficiency. Yet iodine deficiency is still a problem for at least 20% of the world's population, including people in North America who do not use iodised salt.[81,92] Although excess iodine can cause hypothyroidism, an abrupt increase in dietary iodine intake can cause hyperthyroidism. 'Epidemics' of hyperthyroidism have been seen in several countries when iodine was added to the national diet in order to correct widespread iodine deficiency.[78] Hypothyroidism and hyperthyroidism are also known to occur as a result of treatment of heart arrhythmia with amiodarone, an iodine-containing benzofuran.[178] One 100 mg tablet of amiodarone contains 250 times the daily requirement of iodine.[179]

In addition to iodine, iron, selenium and zinc are important for normal thyroid function. Iron deficiency impairs thyroid hormone synthesis by reducing the activity of haem-dependent thyroid peroxidase which iodinates tyrosine residues in Tg.[115] Whereas severe iodine deficiency leads to a neural form of cretinism associated with predominantly neuromotor defects, including strabismus, deaf mutism, spastic diplegia and other disorders of gait and coordination, combined selenium and iodine deficiency leads to a myxoedematous form associated with short stature and markedly delayed bone and sexual maturation, but rarely with deafness or thyroid enlargement.[94] The term 'myxoedema' is derived from the

Greek words *myxa,* meaning 'slime', and *oidema,* meaning 'swelling.' Myxoedema develops after birth and is associated with less severe cerebral deficiency than cretinism. Selenium plays an important role in oxidative defence and intracellular redox regulation and modulation in the body, processes that are thought to be impaired in different types of neurodegenerative diseases, including AD in DS (see below). It is a component of a number of important enzymes, including the glutathione peroxidases which detoxify peroxide, the three deiodinases (D1, D2 and D3) that remove iodide from thyroxine and T3 (thus decreasing the stimulation of oxidative metabolism promoted by thyroxine), the thioredoxine reductases and methionine-sulphoxide reductase.[180] Selenium is incorporated into all of these enzymes in the form of an amino acid to which the selenium is already bound, called selenocysteine.[84]

Thyroid dysfunction is known to influence zinc metabolism, and zinc status in the body is known to influence thyroid function, although the reasons for these effects are not well understood. Zinc may mediate the binding of thyroid hormone receptor to the thyroid hormone response element via its 'zinc fingers.'[84,90] (Zinc fingers are small protein domains in which zinc plays a structural role contributing to the stability of the domains.) Zinc is also a cofactor of cytoplasmic Cu,Zn-superoxide dismutase-1 (SOD1), the enzyme that dismutates superoxide radicals into peroxide in cells[99] (for further information on SOD1 and its possible role in AD in DS, *see* Chapter 5).

Availability of thyroxine-binding proteins

Thyroxine is mostly bound to proteins called thyroxine-binding proteins (TBP). These include thyroxine-binding globulin (TBG), prealbumin (now called trans-thyretin), albumin and apolipoprotein E (ApoE).[89,101] The ApoE gene has three common alleles: ϵ2, ϵ3 and ϵ4. The ϵ4 allele is overexpressed in people with late-onset DAD, yet it is also associated with increased embryo survival.[114] In the Han Chinese, ϵ4 is significantly overexpressed in individuals affected by fetal iodine-deficiency disorder, DAD and vascular dementia.[111,112] This observation suggests an involvement of iodine deficiency and its consequences in all three of these disorders.

Inactivation processes

Once it has exerted its effect, thyroid hormone is inactivated by deiodination and other mechanisms (including glucuronidation, sulphation, oxidative deamination and ether bond cleavage). Three selenium-containing deiodinases (D1, D2 and D3) regulate the levels of T3. In humans, D1 is expressed mainly in liver, kidney and thyroid, D2 is expressed in the brain, pituitary and brown fat, and D3 is restricted to the brain, placenta and pregnant uterus. D1 and D3 deiodinate T4 and T3 and are under positive control by T3. D2 is under negative control by T4, which induces its ubiquitination (addition of ubiquitin groups), accelerating its destruction.[181]

Competition with reverse T3

One derivative of thyroid hormone is called reverse T3 (rT3). This derivative is inactive, but it will compete with T3 for its receptor. The formation of rT3 is promoted by cortisol, the levels of which are increased as a result of stress.[181]

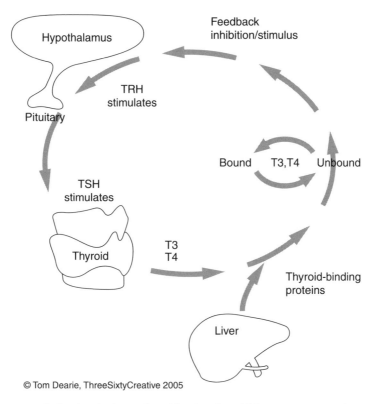

© Tom Dearie, ThreeSixtyCreative 2005

Figure 7.1 Hypothalamic–pituitary–thyroid axis. Thyroid hormones T3 and T4 are controlled by the hypothalamus through a feedback loop. TRH from the hypothalamus triggers T3 and T4 release via TSH from the pituitary. Thyroid-binding proteins then bind circulating T3 and T4. Surplus unbound T3 and T4 inhibit further TRH and TSH release by the hypothalamus and pituitary.

The hypothalamic–pituitary–thyroid axis

The thyroid gland operates in concert with the hypothalamus and the pituitary gland, an arrangement which is referred to as the 'hypothalamic–pituitary–thyroid' (HPT) axis (*see* Figure 7.1). The hypothalamus secretes thyroid-releasing hormone (TRH), which stimulates the anterior pituitary to synthesise and secrete thyrotropin or thyroid-stimulating hormone (TSH). In turn, TSH acts on the thyroid gland to upregulate production of T4 and T3.[106,182]

The HPT axis is subject to feedback inhibition by the circulating thyroid hormones. The synthesis and secretion of TSH are stimulated by TRH in response to low levels of circulating thyroid hormones. T4 and T3 downregulate TSH in a classic feedback inhibition loop. TRH production in the hypothalamus is also inhibited by these thyroid hormones, but to a lesser degree than TSH production. Recently, two other hormones that are produced in the hypothalamus have been shown to affect TSH secretion. Corticotrophin-releasing hormone (CRH), which stimulates the production of adrenocorticotropic hormone (ACTH) by the pituitary, leading to cortisol production by the adrenal glands, has been shown to stimulate TSH secretion. Furthermore, somatostatin blunts the TSH response to TRH and CRH.[86] Primary causes of thyroid dysfunction (i.e. those that directly affect the function of the thyroid gland) are most common. Secondary causes of thyroid dysfunction result from impairment of the function of the hypothalamus or pituitary.[88,100,106,182]

Tests for thyroid function

Normal reference ranges and factors that affect them

Development of the radioimmunoassay in the 1970s revolutionised the study of thyroid hormones and the whole field of endocrinology.[104] It enabled sensitive assays to be developed that are diagnostic for thyroid malfunction. No single laboratory test is 100% accurate in diagnosing all types of thyroid disease. However, a combination of two or more tests usually can be. Table 7.1 lists the tests that are commonly used to assess thyroid function and the representative 'normal' reference ranges in serum samples from adults.

Values for children and for pregnant women are different. Normal ranges from different laboratories will vary slightly, as there is no calibration of the tests between different laboratories.

At present there is concern that normal ranges for most thyroid tests are too broad. This means that certain individuals who are near the upper or lower limits of normal may have some thyroid malfunction. There are several reasons why normal ranges for thyroid tests may be too broad. Test results are known to be affected by genetic factors, time of day and season of the year, age, gender and

Table 7.1 Typical serum reference ranges for thyroid tests in adults aged 20–80 years

Test	Normal reference range
TSH	0.5–5 µU/ml
Total T4 (TT4)	5.0–12.0 g/dl or 64.4–154.4 nmol/l
Free T4	0.9–2.0 ng/dl or 12–26 pmol/l
Free T4 index (T7 or FT4I) (total T4 × T3 uptake)	5–12 SI units
Total T3 (TT3)	95–200 ng/dl or 1.5–3.0 nmol/l
Free T3	0.2–0.52 ng/dl or 3–8 pmol/l
Free T3 index (FT3I)	1.3–4.2 or 16–54 SI units
T3 uptake (indirect measure of thyroid-binding globulins)	23–35% or 0.2–0.35 SI units
Thyroid antibodies (to thyroglobulin, peroxidase, thyroid receptor)	Values differ between laboratories
Other (iodine uptake scan, thyroid scans, ultrasound, needle biopsy)	

Thyroid hormone tests. Normal reference ranges; www.keratin.com/ab/ab011.shtml#03.[109]

probably fasting, but such factors are not usually taken into consideration when normal ranges are established. When people are tested on more than one occasion, inter-individual variation in serum TSH, free T4 and free T3 concentrations has been found to be much greater than intra-individual variation, which suggests that each individual may have a genetically determined thyroid function set-point.[15,79,80,104,105,183]

Thyroid function tests and interpretation

Thyroid-stimulating hormone (TSH)

Normally, low levels (less than 3–5 units) of TSH are sufficient to keep the normal thyroid gland functioning properly. Clinically, measurement of the serum TSH level is used first to assess thyroid status. An elevated TSH level is indicative of primary hypothyroidism, whereas a lowered level is indicative of primary hyperthyroidism. The first-generation TSH tests had no lower limit of normal. The second- and third-generation tests have clearly defined lower limits, and involve the use of two or more antibodies directed to different portions of TSH.[107,117]

Thyroid hormones

Measurements of T4 and T3 levels aid the diagnosis of thyroid status. Elevated T4 levels are characteristically seen in patients with primary hyperthyroidism, whereas T4 levels are generally reduced in patients with primary hypothyroidism. Normal T4 levels accompanied by high T3 values are seen in patients with *T3 thyrotoxicosis*. Thyroxine levels may be altered by physiological or pathological changes in TBP capacity. Drugs that compete for T4-binding sites in the T4 assay, such as phenylbutazone, diphenylhydantoin or salicylates, can result in a lowered T4 measurement. Serum T4 levels in neonates and infants are higher than the corresponding values in the normal adult, due to the increased concentration of TBG in neonate serum. Thyroxine values should therefore be normalised for variation in TBP capacity. The free thyroxine index (FT4I) is used to achieve this measurement.[101,103,104,106]

The following serum tests are commonly used to characterise thyroid hormone function.[104,106,108]

- **Total T4.** This represents the total amount of T4. Uncorrected T4 levels may be high not only as a result of hyperthyroidism, but also due to pregnancy, oral contraceptive pills, oestrogen replacement therapy and other factors.
- **Free T4.** This test directly measures the free T4 level in the blood.
- **Total T3.** This test is usually ordered when thyroid disease is being investigated. T3 is more potent and short-lived than T4. Some people with an overactive thyroid secrete more T3 than T4. In such cases, T4 levels can be normal, T3 levels elevated and TSH levels low. Total T3 is a measure of the total amount of T3 in the bloodstream, including the T3 bound to carrier proteins plus free and circulating T3.
- **Free T3.** This measures only the T3 that is free and not bound to carrier proteins.
- **T3 resin uptake.** This is not a thyroid test. It reflects the level of proteins that carry thyroid hormone in the bloodstream. A high T3 resin uptake level reflects a low level of these proteins.

- **Free thyroxine index.** A mathematical computation allows the laboratory to estimate the free thyroxine index from the T4 and T3 uptake tests. The result indicates how much thyroid hormone is freely available in the body.

Thyroid antibodies

Some individuals produce antibodies to thyroglobulin, thyroid peroxidase or the TSH receptor. The measurement of titres of thyroid autoantibodies should be undertaken if the TSH is mildly abnormal but T4 and T3 indicators are normal.[104,106,108]

Abnormalities of thyroid function

Thyroid dysfunction in the general population

Prevalence rates of thyroid disorders vary markedly from one country to another, but they generally show increasing frequency with age and they also occur more commonly in women. About one in 13 people (7.35%) in the USA have diagnosed thyroid disorders, and about one in 20 (4.78%) have undiagnosed thyroid disease.[128] Low-grade functional disorders are more common than cases of overt disease.

Hyperthyroidism

A laboratory diagnosis of hyperthyroidism is characterised by the following:

- decreased TSH and elevated T4 (primary)
- elevated T4/T3, FT4I and TSH (secondary and tertiary).

The prevalence of hyperthyroidism in community-based studies in the USA has been estimated to be 2% for women and 0.2% for men. As many as 15% of cases of hyperthyroidism occur in patients over 60 years of age.[184] There are several causes of hyperthyroidism. Most often the entire gland is overproducing thyroid hormone. This is called Graves' disease. Less commonly, a single nodule is responsible for the excess hormone secretion. This is referred to as a 'hot' nodule. Inflammation of the thyroid gland, known as thyroiditis, can lead to the release of excess amounts of thyroid hormones. Hyperthyroidism can also occur in patients who are taking excessive doses of any of the available forms of thyroid hormone.

Clinical manifestations of hyperthyroidism include weight loss, loss of muscle mass, dyspnoea, loss of fat stores, exercise intolerance, easy fatiguability, nervousness, irritability, insomnia, tremor, heat intolerance, excessive sweating, increased cardiac output, diarrhoea, changes in menstrual periods and warm moist skin.[123] A disorder dubbed 'apathetic hyperthyroidism' (paradoxical presentation of hyperthyroidism with fatigue, psychomotor slowing, depression and weight gain) is common in the elderly.[29] This condition can exacerbate chronic diseases, especially cardiovascular conditions.

Hypothyroidism

A laboratory diagnosis of hypothyroidism is characterised by the following:

- increased TSH and decreased T4 (primary)
- decreased T4, T3, FT4I and TSH (secondary and tertiary).

This disorder is associated with the presence of insufficient thyroid hormones to meet metabolic needs. It may be congenital (i.e. present since birth, transient or permanent) or acquired.

Congenital hypothyroidism
This disorder occurs when the thyroid gland fails to develop or function properly. In 80–85% of cases the thyroid gland is absent, abnormally located or severely reduced in size. In the remaining cases, a normal-sized or enlarged thyroid gland is present, but production of thyroid hormones is decreased or absent. Although many countries have introduced programmes to prevent iodine deficiency by providing iodised salt, fetal iodine deficiency is still the commonest cause of congenital hypothyroidism worldwide, affecting as many as 10% of individuals in an iodine-deficient area. Worldwide, the frequency of congenital hypothyroidism resulting from iodine deficiency is about 18 in 1000.[95–97] If babies with iodine deficiency are not treated, cretinism will develop (see above).

In iodine-replete areas, the incidence of congenital hypothyroidism from other causes ranges from about 1 in 3000 to 1 in 4000.[116,185] Congenital hypothyroidism with a genetic basis occurs sporadically in about 85% of cases. Mutations in the following genes are now known to cause congenital hypothyroidism that is not a result of iodine deficiency: PAX8 (essential for regulation of the thyroglobulin gene by transforming growth factor); SLC5A5 (provides instructions for synthesising a protein that facilitates the uptake of iodide in certain tissues); Tg; thyroid peroxidase (TPO); thyroid-synthesising hormone β-subunit (TSHB); thyroid-synthesising hormone receptor (TSHR). Mutations in other genes that have not yet been well characterised may also cause congenital hypothyroidism.[120] Gene mutations cause the loss of thyroid function in one of two ways. Mutations in the PAX8 gene and some mutations in the TSHR gene prevent or disrupt the development of the thyroid gland before birth. Mutations in the SLC5A5, Tg, TPO and TSHB genes prevent or reduce the production of thyroid hormones, even though the thyroid gland is present. If treatment for congenital hypothyroidism is started within a month after birth, children develop almost normally. However, because they still undergo a brief period of thyroid hormone deficiency, they are at risk for subtle selective impairments.[185] As neuropsychological tools have become more sensitive, it has become apparent that even mild thyroid hormone deficiency in humans can produce measurable deficits in very specific neuropsychological functions. Interestingly, among newborns in the general population who have been diagnosed with congenital hypothyroidism, there is evidence for an unusually high frequency of other congenital birth defects, including cardiac anomalies and gastrointestinal anomalies, raising the possibility that multiple congenital anomalies in single individuals have resulted from the same teratogenic event.[186,187]

Acquired overt hypothyroidism
The overall prevalence of overt hypothyroidism in the USA is 5–10 in 1000 in the general population. Above the age of 65 years it increases to 6–10% of women and 2–3% of men. It occurs more frequently in women than in men (female:male ratio, 5–10:1). As many as 3–5% of the population are thought to have some degree of hypothyroidism. Some of the common causes of hypothyroidism include Hashimoto's thyroiditis, lymphocytic thyroiditis, thyroid destruction,

hypothalmic or pituitary disease, pituitary injury, medications and iodine deficiency.[78,106]

Overt hypothyroidism in adults is associated with a familiar set of symptoms and signs, including fatigue, weakness, weight gain or difficulty losing weight, slowed heart rate, coarse dry hair, dry rough pale skin, hair loss, cold intolerance, muscle cramps, frequent muscle aches, constipation, irritability, memory loss or slowed mental processing, abnormal menstrual cycles and decreased libido. However, such symptoms cannot be used to reliably diagnose hypothyroidism. Once a diagnosis has been made on the basis of quantitative laboratory measurements, treatment is straightforward and the patient's prognosis is excellent.[124] A normal TSH level does not exclude central hypothyroidism involving hypothalamic or pituitary dysfunction, which may not be as rare in elderly people as was previously thought.[29]

Autoimmune thyroiditis

This disorder is characterised by elevated titres of autoantibodies produced against TSH, thyroid peroxidase or the TSH receptor. Autoimmune thyroiditis may or may not be accompanied by altered levels of TSH or the thyroid hormones. Graves' disease, Hashimoto's thyroiditis and Ord's thyroiditis are examples of autoimmune thyroid disorders termed 'autoimmune thyroiditis.' Interestingly, Hashimoto's thyroiditis is associated with goitre (enlargement of the thyroid gland), whereas Ord's thyroiditis is associated with thyroid atrophy. Hashimoto's thyroiditis is reported to be common in North America, whereas Ord's thyroiditis occurs more frequently than Hashimoto's in Europe.[188] De Quervain's thyroiditis (also called subacute or granulomatous thyroiditis) is much less common than Hashimoto's thyroiditis. The thyroid gland generally swells rapidly and is very painful and tender. The gland discharges thyroid hormone into the blood and the patient becomes hyperthyroid. However, the gland stops taking up iodine and the hyperthyroidism generally resolves over the next few weeks. Silent thyroiditis is the least common type of thyroiditis. The majority of patients with the latter disorder are young women following pregnancy. The disease usually requires no treatment, and 80% of patients show complete recovery, with the thyroid gland returning to normal after about three months.[78,107,188]

It is not known whether antithyroid antibodies cause thyroid disease, whether thyroid disease causes the antibodies, or whether the antibodies' functions are physiologically beneficial.[127] Rarely, elderly people with autoimmune hypothyroidism have a condition called Hashimoto's encephalopathy, which features cognitive abnormalities (usually a delirium state but sometimes a stroke-like syndrome).[65] Thyroid hormones are unlikely to be directly involved in this condition, which may respond to corticosteroid treatment.

Euthyroid 'sick syndrome'

This term refers to abnormalities in thyroid function that are not caused by primary thyroid or pituitary dysfunction.[87] Causes are thought to include hypothalamic and pituitary suppression, decreased conversion of T4 to T3, alterations in serum binding of thyroid hormones, and decreased TSH production and/or its effect on the thyroid. Cytokines such as tumour necrosis factor alpha, interleukin-1, interleukin-6, free fatty acids, cortisol and glucagon all have effects on thyroid function. Abnormalities of thyroid function also result from conditions such as surgical stress and serious infection. It is not clear whether these changes reflect a protective response in the face of a serious illness, or a maladaptive process that needs to be corrected. Some patterns of abnormalities that fall into the category of euthyroid 'sick syndrome' include the following.

- **Low T3 with an increase in rT3.** This is thought to be due to a decrease in the conversion of T4 to T3 by the hepatic deiodinase system.
- **Low T3 and low T4 with normal to low TSH.** This may be due to low TBG levels or the presence of a thyroid-hormone-binding inhibitor.
- **Low TSH, low T3 and low T4.** This suggests an alteration in pituitary or hypothalamic responsiveness.
- **Elevated T4 with normal or elevated TSH and normal or elevated T3.** This may be seen in primary biliary cirrhosis and acute or chronic hepatitis in which TBG synthesis and release are increased, in acute psychiatric illnesses, and as a result of use of certain drugs.[83,106]

Thyroid dysfunction in Down syndrome

History

The first suggestion of a link between thyroid dysfunction and DS was made unintentionally over 130 years ago before the disorder of DS had been formally recognised. In 1866, a French physician, Edouard Seguin, described a condition termed 'furfuraceous' cretinism in a particular subgroup of children:

> With its milk-white, rosy, and peeling skin; with its shortcomings of all the integuments, which give an unfinished aspect to the truncated fingers and nose; with its cracked lips and tongue; with its red, ectopic conjunctiva, coming out to supply the curtailed skin at the margin of the lids.[22]

Retrospectively, some people have suspected that 'furfuraceous cretinism' was in fact the disorder now known as DS, although there is not universal agreement about this.

In 1866, John Langdon Haydon Down coined the term 'mongoloid' to denote the characteristics of a group of children with the remarkably similar abnormalities that we now associate with DS, and to distinguish such abnormalities from those in cretinism.[119] Before the genetic reason for DS was known, many people thought that the syndrome was caused by hypothyroidism. One reason for this was that, in 1896, Telford Smith reported that giving thyroid therapy improved the physical and mental condition of these children.[23] Another reason was that two autopsy studies revealed a high rate of thyroid abnormality in 'mongolism.' One study, published in 1903, reported that all thyroid glands were histopathologically abnormal in these individuals.[3] A second study, published in 1948, reported that only one out of 48 thyroid glands examined was normal, 20% having colloidal goitre with scattered areas of hyperplasia.[1,11] Although these fascinating studies suggest that the thyroid gland may be morphologically abnormal in all people with DS, they should be treated with caution because it was not until the 1970s that an objective distinction could be made between DS and cretinism.[18] A definite diagnosis of DS became possible in 1959 when Jerome Lejeune and Patricia Jacobs independently discovered that people with the clinical phenotype of DS carried an extra chromosome, which is now called chromosome 21.[189,190] With the advent of the radioimmunoassay in the 1970s that led to accurate measurement of thyroid hormones in blood, it became possible to categorise thyroid disorders and to make an objective distinction between conditions of overt thyroid dysfunction and DS. However, clinical laboratory testing has revealed an unusually high frequency of clinically abnormal thyroid results in individuals with DS, the majority being indicative of subclinical hypothyroidism (see below).

Thyroid abnormalities occur in all age groups in DS.[4,8,9,11,15,129] Clinical forms of hypothyroidism that are found in individuals with DS include congenital hypothyroidism, transient and primary hypothyroidism, compensated hypothyroidism, pituitary–hypothalamic hypothyroidism, TBG deficiency, autoimmune thyroiditis and chronic lymphocytic thyroiditis. Hyperthyroidism also occurs. As in the general population,[187,191] babies with congenital hypothyroidism and DS are at increased risk of having other congenital abnormalities. In one study, congenital hypothyroidism in DS was found to occur significantly more frequently in individuals diagnosed with congenital gastrointestinal anomalies than in those without such a diagnosis.[192] Thyroid disease is difficult to diagnose clinically in individuals with DS because of the overlap of symptoms. This means that thyroid blood screening is a particularly important part of the annual preventive medicine screening of each person with DS.

When data from thyroid function tests are compared in newborns with or without DS, there is evidence that a high percentage of newborns with DS have abnormalities in thyroid function, in particular somewhat elevated TSH levels and somewhat reduced T4 levels.[26] Because newborns with DS are rarely treated for thyroid problems, an important question is whether some of the characteristics attributed to DS, such as impairment of development and growth, may be the result of neonatal thyroid dysfunction. Van Trotsenburg and colleagues[26] conducted a single-centre, randomised, double-blind, 24-month trial with nationwide recruitment, comparing thyroxine administration with placebo in 196 neonates with DS in order to address this issue. Compared with placebo, thyroxine treatment significantly reduced the delay in motor development and mental development in the study population. Furthermore, children who were treated with thyroxine were taller and heavier than those who were not treated. This study concluded that thyroxine treatment of neonates with DS should be considered in order to maximise their development and growth. However, the long-term consequences of thyroid hormone treatment need to be considered. Unnecessary treatment with thyroid hormone can lead to bone demineralisation and cardiac arrhythmias.[11] Furthermore, *in-vitro* and *in-vivo* studies indicate that thyroid hormones have a strong influence on oxidative stress, a state that develops when antioxidative defence mechanisms are not sufficient to cope with cellular damage resulting from oxidative processes.[163]

Thyroid dysfunction in adults with Down syndrome

A number of papers have covered the topic of thyroid dysfunction in adults with DS.[5,6,11–13,15,17–20,25–27] There is an age effect on the frequency of thyroid abnormalities in individuals with DS as well as in the general population, the frequency increasing with age. Autoimmune thyroiditis associated with mild hypothyroidism is very common, with as many as 30% of people over the age of 40 years being affected. Males as well as females with DS are prone to developing thyroid dysfunction, although the frequency is higher in females. Overt hypothyroidism and overt hyperthyroidism are also more common in adults with DS than in the general population.[9,15]

An important issue that needs to be further investigated is whether the apparently increased prevalence of mild hypothyroidism in adults with DS results artefactually from the use of reference ranges for people without DS.[19] It has been argued that if reference ranges for healthy people with DS are used, prevalence rates for hypothyroidism would be the same as in the general population. On the other hand, the increased prevalence of thyroid dysfunction in individuals with DS may reflect accelerated ageing and/or early onset of DAD in this population.[15,19] The finding of abnormal histopathology in the thyroid glands of individuals with DS, and the striking association of autoimmune thyroiditis in older people with DS with the HLA DQA 0301 antigen[13] and with chronic hepatitis B virus infection,[12] support the hypothesis that the high frequency of thyroid disorders in DS is not entirely a result of using inappropriate reference ranges. Other reported associations with apparent thyroid dysfunction in DS include the following:

- a statistical association between elevated TSH levels and the presence of autoantibodies to gliadin (characteristic of coeliac disease)[24]
- an association between elevated TSH levels and lowered serum selenium levels[7]
- among females with DS, an association between treated hypothyroidism and the ϵ4 allele of ApoE, the ϵ2 allele appearing to be protective[16]
- a possible association between hypothyroidism and arthritic presentations in DS.[2]

Interestingly, having DS may protect against the development of malignant neoplasms of the thyroid.[21] Some key findings with regard to thyroid dysfunction in adults with DS are listed in Table 7.2.

Subclinical hypothyroidism in the general population and in individuals with Down syndrome

Subclinical hypothyroidism is defined as elevated TSH with normal thyroxine levels, or normal TSH with low thyroxine levels. Because the laboratory reference ranges are so broad, individuals whose test results fall just within the current normal limits may have mild thyroid disease. An issue that is currently controversial is whether or not people with subclinical thyroid disease, especially subclinical hypothyroidism, should be treated.[133]

On the one hand, it is possible that even slightly abnormal thyroid hormone results may affect cognitive function. For example, in a study of 628 women aged 65 years or over who were community based and physically impaired, the relationship between cognitive function and levels of thyroid hormones was assessed at entry to the study and after 1, 2 and 3 years, using the Mini Mental State Examination.[134] Although no association between T4 and TSH levels and cognitive function was noted at the start of the study, those women with the lowest levels of thyroid hormones had a twofold higher risk of cognitive decline,

Table 7.2 Some key findings with regard to thyroid dysfunction in adults with Down syndrome

Study	Findings
Percy et al. (1990)[15]	Autoimmune thyroiditis associated with mild, subclinical hypothyroidism was found to be common in older people with DS. This disorder was found to affect more people and to be milder in DS than the hypothyroidism that affects older people in the general population. Compared with healthy control individuals without DS or ID, patients with DS had, overall, lower mean total T4 and free T3, higher T3U and TSH, no difference in free T4, and higher thyroid antithyroglobulin and antimicrosomal autoantibody titres. Similar trends were apparent in males and females with DS, and in individuals with DS who were not taking any drugs
Hestnes et al. (1991)[6]	Clinical and laboratory endocrine variables in adult institutionalised patients with DS were compared with those for matched controls consisting of other patients with ID from the same institution. The average TSH level in DS patients was higher than in the controls. There was no clear-cut correlation between TSH and thyroid hormone levels. The data indicated a tendency towards primary thyroid dysfunction in DS. There was some evidence of a relative failure of TSH secretion
Nicholson et al. (1994)[13]	Susceptibility to autoimmune thyroiditis in DS was found to be associated with the major histocompatibility class II DQA 0301 allele
May and Kawanishi (1996)[12]	The frequency of thyroiditis in patients with DS who were also carriers of hepatitis B virus surface antigen (HBsAg) was threefold higher than the frequency of thyroiditis in those patients with DS who were not carriers of HBsAg (65% vs. 23%; $P < 0.01$). No similar association was observed in patients with ID who did not have DS
Storm (1996)[24]	A statistical correlation was found between increased TSH levels and a positive titre for gliadin antibodies, which are characteristic of coeliac disease in DS
Rooney and Walsh (1997)[20]	Abnormalities in thyroid function tests were found to occur more frequently in patients with DS who were institutionalised than in those who lived in the community
Kanavin et al. (2000)[7]	Increased TSH, decreased free T4 and decreased serum selenium levels were found in institutionalised adults with DS compared with people with ID matched for age, gender and behavioural function as controls. A positive correlation was observed between serum concentrations of free T4 and selenium in the patients with DS ($r = 0.393$, $P < 0.05$)

Table 7.2 (*cont.*)

Study	Findings
Percy *et al.* (2003)[16]	In older women with DS, there was an ApoE allele effect on thyroid status, with $\epsilon2$ negatively ($P \leq 0.01$) and $\epsilon4$ positively ($P \leq 0.05$) associated with treated hypothyroidism. In this case hypothyroidism was defined as having at least one elevated serum TSH level. There was no evidence for an ApoE allele effect on thyroid status in older men with DS
Bosch *et al.* (2004)[2]	Among eight patients with DS who had a slipped capital femoral epiphysis, hypothyroidism was diagnosed in 6 cases. This observation raised the possibility that hypothyroidism is a predisposing factor for this disorder, at least in DS
Prasher and Haque (2004)[19]	About one-third of a group of apparently healthy adults with DS were found to have subclinical hypothyroidism (elevated TSH with normal free T4 or low free T4 with normal TSH levels). The others were biochemically euthyroid. The authors raised the question of whether standard general population laboratory free T4 and TSH reference ranges are really applicable to the DS population. They pointed out that adults with DS are susceptible to premature ageing, and that the higher TSH values might reflect this. They also pointed out that use of the current standard laboratory reference ranges for thyroid function tests does not allow researchers or physicians to take an age effect into account
Satge *et al.* (2004)[21]	Malignant neoplasia of the thyroid were found to be rare in DS

leading the authors to conclude that low thyroid hormone levels may contribute to cognitive impairment in physically impaired women.[134] In another study of 36 older women with mild hypothyroidism, Bono and colleagues[130] found an improvement in verbal fluency and depression scores, and a positive correlation between TSH reduction and improved mood scores after treatment with L-thyroxine, supporting the treatment of asymptomatic mild hypothyroidism in order to reset hormonal levels and protect the brain against the potential risk of cognitive and affective dysfunction. Yet in population studies of the 'oldest old', subclinical hypothyroidism was not associated with adverse health effects, and was in fact associated with a survival advantage.[131–133]

This issue of whether or not to treat subclinical hypothyroidism is even more relevant in the case of people with DS. As already mentioned, hypothyroidism appears to be greatly over-represented in this disorder, affecting as many as 30–50% of DS patients in their lifetime.[9,15] In particular, in early infancy as many as 80–90% of neonates with DS appear to have mild hypothyroidism.[26] The cause(s) of subclinical disease in people with DS is not known. It may be due to a true thyroid hormone deficiency and a consequence of trisomy 21 itself, or it may be due to a micronutrient deficiency (e.g. iodine, selenium or zinc deficiency) or other causes (see summary and discussion). Alternatively, as already discussed, subclinical hypothyroidism may be at least in part an artefact resulting from the use of reference ranges for people without DS.[19] Furthermore, it has yet to be established whether there are different causes of subclinical thyroid abnormalities in individuals with DS over their lifespan. In conclusion, well-designed clinical trials are needed to determine the advantages and/or disadvantages of treating very mild abnormalities of thyroid function in DS patients as well as in the general population.

Thyroid dysfunction and dementia in Alzheimer's disease

Rationale for a possible connection

For many years there has been considerable interest in the hypothesis that thyroid dysfunction is an integral feature of AD. If thyroid status or levels of thyroid hormones are consistently abnormal in a high percentage of patients with DAD, then such measurements might be used as diagnostic markers for DAD in the general population. Some reasons that have fuelled studies in this area include the following:

- Some cases of dementia are known to be the result of hypothyroidism caused by thyroid hormone deficiency. If the hypothyroidism is treated at an early stage, it can often be reversed.[28,29,31] When dementia is first diagnosed, efforts should be directed towards ruling out the presence of thyroid hormone deficiency, and at least nine other disorders that are potentially reversible.[29] As discussed above, even very mild hypothyroidism may have an effect on cognitive function.
- A high percentage of people worldwide suffer from iodine deficiency and are therefore prone to developing clinical thyroid dysfunction.[118] Iodine deficiency may result in hypothyroidism that is overt or subclinical,[97] and such deficiency has been implicated theoretically in AD and in Parkinson's disease.[37]
- It has been proposed that thyroid hormone deficiency in the central nervous system, resulting from a variety of causes, including insufficient blood flow to the brain, may cause or contribute to DAD.[60]
- Brain changes occur in AD that may affect thyroid function. Neuropathological studies of adults in the general population with DAD, and of adults with DS and DAD, have demonstrated that neurochemical changes occur not only in the cerebral cortex but also in the hypothalamus, which is involved in the regulation of thyroid hormone production. Characteristic neurochemical changes include a reduction in choline acetyltransferase activity.[193–197] Because the somatostatinergic system inhibits the release of TSH, a decrease in somatostatin levels would result in an increase in TSH levels.[198] Loss of brain tissue as a result of neurodegeneration may also affect the function of the HPT axis in people with DAD.

Other observations that support the involvement of thyroid function in AD are listed in Table 7.3. Of particular interest are the effects of thyroid hormone on the expression of choline acetyltransferase[59] and also on the expression of APP and its splice variants.[52,72] (Choline acetyltransferase is the enzyme that catalyses the formation of acetylcholine, levels of which are reduced in AD. Deposits of

Table 7.3 *In-vitro* studies that support the possible involvement of thyroid function in dementia or Alzheimer's disease

Study	Findings
Sutherland *et al.* (1992)[68]	Message levels for a thyroid hormone receptor located on chromosome 21 and highly expressed in brain (c-ERB A alpha) were reduced by 52% in CA1 and 43% in CA2 in AD hippocampus compared with Huntington controls
Benvenga *et al.* (1993)[136]	Exon 3 of ApoE was found to carry a thyroid-hormone-binding domain (the ε4 allele of ApoE is a major risk factor for DAD; the binding of thyroid hormone to different ApoE isoforms may vary)
Quirin-Stricker *et al.* (1994)[59]	Thyroid hormone activates the human choline acetyltransferase gene via binding of thyroid hormone receptor to its 5′ untranslated region
Schmitt *et al.* (1995)[62]	Thyroid epithelial cells were found to produce large amounts of the Alzheimer β-APP and potentially amyloidogenic APP fragments
Schmitt *et al.* (1996)[63]	The production of an amyloidogenic metabolite of APP in thyroid cells was found to be stimulated by interleukin-1-β, but inhibited by interferon-γ
Belandia *et al.* (1998)[30]	Thyroid hormone was found to negatively regulate the transcriptional activity of the β-APP gene
Latasa *et al.* (1998)[52]	Thyroid hormones were found to regulate β-amyloid gene splicing and protein secretion in neuroblastoma cells
Labudova *et al.* (1999)[51]	TSH receptor was found to be overexpressed in the brains of patients with DS and DAD
Luo *et al.* (2002)[57]	Decreased thyrotropin-releasing hormone levels were found in the hippocampus of patients with DAD compared with normal controls
Villa *et al.* (2004)[72]	A response unit in the first exon of the β-APP gene containing thyroid hormone receptor and Sp1 binding sites was found to mediate negative regulation by T3

amyloid β-peptide (Aβ), a breakdown product of APP, are a characteristic hallmark of AD; *see* Chapter 1.)

Association between thyroid disease and Alzheimer's disease in the general population

For the general population, a considerable number of clinical studies have investigated an association between thyroid disease and DAD (*see* Table 7.4). The first such studies were reported by Heyman and colleagues, who investigated genetic aspects and a number of possible associated clinical disorders in 68 adults in whom dementia appeared before the age of 70 years.[45,46] Although the studies primarily focused on DAD presenting in the relatives of individuals with familial DAD, they did show that of the 68 probands, 14 individuals (one man and 13

Table 7.4 Studies that have investigated a clinical association between thyroid disease and Alzheimer's disease in the general population

Study	Findings
Heyman et al. (1983, 1984)[45,46]	History of thyroid disease was found to be significantly more frequent in DAD probands than in non-DAD controls
Small et al. (1985)[64]	No significant association between DAD and thyroid dysfunction was found in individuals with DAD
Tappy et al. (1987)[69]	Hypothyroidism was not found to be significantly associated with cognitive disorders
Lawlor et al. (1988)[53]	No significant difference in history of thyroid disease was found between DAD and non-DAD subjects
Katzman et al. (1989)[50]	Risk factors for DAD were investigated, and thyroid disease was not found to be a significant risk factor
Lopez et al. (1989)[55]	Findings did not support an association between thyroid disorders and DAD
Yoshimasu et al. (1991)[77]	For myxoedema, there was a positive non-significant association with DAD. For Graves' disease, there was a statistically significant negative association with DAD
Edwards et al. (1991)[34]	The frequency of thyroid dysfunction was found to be similar in individuals with familial and non-familial DAD
Lopez et al. (2000)[56]	The authors examined the clinical characteristics of 267 patients diagnosed with possible DAD. They identified six categories of patients: possible DAD with cerebrovascular disease (69%), with history of alcohol abuse (15%), with history of depression (7%), with thyroid disease (4%), with history of head trauma (6%), with vitamin B_{12} deficiency (6%), and with other disease processes that may have affected the clinical presentation of DAD (4%). Thus thyroid disease is not a major factor in DAD

women) had a history of thyroid disease or were receiving thyroid hormone replacement therapy. This number was significantly more than expected. A significantly higher frequency of previous thyroid disease was found in female patients than in female control subjects (25% and 7.1%, respectively), and a possible association between DAD and thyroid dysfunction was highlighted.

Although thyroid dysfunction can occur concurrently with DAD, most population studies conducted subsequent to the reports of Heyman and colleagues have failed to confirm a significant excess of thyroid disease in patients with DAD compared with a non-DAD control group.[34,64,69] However, Yoshimasu and colleagues found a trend towards a positive association of myxoedema with DAD and a statistically significant negative association of Graves' disease with DAD.[77] In conclusion, the above data indicate that comorbid overt thyroid disease does exist in a relatively small percentage of patients with DAD, but that it is not a major factor in AD.

Association between thyroid dysfunction and dementia in Alzheimer's disease in the general population

Rather than investigating the association between thyroid dysfunction and DAD, a number of researchers have investigated the possibility that abnormalities in the levels of thyroid hormone in serum, plasma or cerebrospinal fluid could be used as markers for DAD (*see* Table 7.5). Although some studies have reported negative or non-significant results, others have reported positive findings. Furthermore, in studies of individuals with DAD, hypothyroidism and hyperthyroidism have been observed. Although the published data document thyroid dysfunction in DAD, it is unclear whether abnormalities of thyroid function are useful markers for DAD.

Association between thyroid hormone dysfunction and dementia in Alzheimer's disease in Down syndrome

A limited number of studies on the association between thyroid hormone dysfunction, cognitive dysfunction and/or DAD have been reported for the DS population.[15–17,73,74,75] As in the general population, conflicting results have been found. Percy and colleagues investigated thyroid disorder in adults with DS and DAD.[15] A total of 46 individuals with DS (community and institution based) were recruited, of mean age 45.3 years (range 31–70 years), as well as 36 age-matched healthy controls. The individuals with DS were divided into those with probable dementia and those without the condition, using the guidelines of MacKhann and colleagues.[76] Compared with healthy controls, the DS group as a whole had lower mean total T4 and T3 levels. In this study it was not possible to age-match individuals with DS and dementia to those without dementia, as individuals who showed manifestations of dementia were significantly older than those who did not. When corrections were applied for age and gender, individuals with DS and DAD had significantly lower T3 levels compared with individuals with DS without manifestations of DAD. The authors concluded that there was an association between mild 'subclinical' hypothyroidism and DAD in the DS population.

Bhaumik and colleagues[73] published evidence that mild hypothyroidism might be protective in DS and that more severe hypothyroidism might be harmful. They demonstrated in a group of 26 institutionalised DS patients with normal thyroid function that global scores of ability (assessed by using Part 1 of the Adaptive Behavior Scale (ABS)) were higher than those in a group of patients with elevated TSH levels in the presence of normal T3 and T4 levels. The actual concentration of TSH was shown to be significantly and inversely related to the score for global abilities. The authors suggested that estimation of TSH levels might provide confirmatory evidence of clinical dementia in people with DS.

Prasher[17] investigated the association between thyroid dysfunction (as indicated by T4 and TSH levels) and DAD in 201 adults with DS, of whom 27 subjects fulfilled the *ICD–10* criteria for DAD.[199] Nine out of 26 demented individuals (34.5%) for whom data on thyroid status were available had thyroid dysfunction, compared with 41 out of 116 non-demented subjects (35.3%). No statistically significant difference was found between the two groups.

Devenny and colleagues[74] monitored groups of adults with or without DS and mild or moderate mental retardation over a six-year period on yearly measures of

Table 7.5 Clinical studies investigating a biochemical association between thyroid dysfunction and dementia, including Alzheimer's disease, in the general population

Study	Findings
Sunderland et al. (1985)[67]	Baseline TSH, total T4 and free T4 levels were higher in DAD than in non-DAD subjects. DAD subjects showed a blunting of the TSH response to the TRH stimulation test
Christie et al. (1987)[32]	Statistically significantly higher plasma levels of TSH were found in patients with DAD than in controls
Thomas et al. (1987)[70]	Compared with controls, the DAD group had significantly lower plasma T3 levels but showed no difference in T4 and T3 levels
Ichibangase et al. (1990)[47]	Cognitive function was found to be closely related to serum free T3 levels and cardiac function in subjects with cerebrovascular dementia. It was concluded that serum free T3 concentrations may be a good indicator of health and cognitive status
Molchan et al. (1991)[58]	DAD patients with a blunted TSH response had significantly higher mean free T4 levels ($P < 0.03$) and tended to be more severely demented than those with a non-blunted response
Faldt et al. (1996)[36]	No significant association was found between thyroid dysfunction and DAD
Ganguli et al. (1996)[39]	A significant association was found between elevated TSH levels and definite dementia, as well as possible and/or definite dementia, in a community-based sample. The findings are consistent with the hypothesis that subclinical hypothyroidism is associated with cognitive impairment and that thyroid state may influence cerebral metabolism
Kalmijn et al. (2000)[48]	Subclinical hyperthyroidism in the elderly was found to be associated with an increased risk of DAD. Individuals with reduced TSH levels at baseline had a more than threefold increased risk of dementia, after adjustment for age and gender. Among individuals with reduced TSH levels, T4 levels appeared to be positively related to the risk of dementia, although none of those who became demented had a T4 level above the normal range. The risk of dementia was markedly increased in subjects with low TSH levels who were positive for TPO-Abs (relative risk = 23.7)
Kapaki et al. (2003)[49]	Cholinesterase inhibitors used to treat DAD were found to produce significant changes in free T3 levels as a function of duration of treatment. Free T3 levels were significantly higher in patients who received cholinesterase treatment for 6–12 months, but then decreased
Dobert et al. (2003)[33]	Decreased or borderline TSH values were found to be associated with an increased probability of having dementia, especially vascular dementia

Table 7.5 (*cont.*)

Study	Findings
Spiegel *et al.* (2004)[65]	Two patients with a syndrome consisting of rapidly progressive dementia with myoclonus were found to have Hashimoto's encephalopathy
Van Osch *et al.* (2004)[71]	In a study of DAD patients and cognitively screened control subjects who were all euthyroid, lowered TSH levels within the normal range were found to be a risk factor for DAD, independent of several cerebrovascular risk factors and confounding variables
Sampaolo *et al.* (2005)[61]	In a study of the cerebrospinal fluid of euthyroid patients with overt DAD and matched healthy controls, DAD subjects showed significantly increased rT(3) levels and an increased ratio of rT(3) to T(4) in the face of unchanged cerebrospinal fluid total T(4) and transthyretin levels. These results suggest that there is abnormal intracerebral thyroid hormone metabolism and possibly brain hypothyroidism, either as a secondary consequence of the ongoing process or as a cofactor in the progression of the disease

mental status, short- and long-term memory, speed of psychomotor function and visuospatial organisation. Only four out of the 91 individuals with DS in their current sample showed changes in functioning that led to a diagnosis of possible DAD, and in these individuals causes of decline in performance other than DAD were concurrently present (e.g. thyroid dysfunction). These findings indicate that some age-associated changes in functioning are related to 'normal' but probably precocious ageing in adults with DS. Furthermore, these results suggest that adults with DS and mild or moderate mental retardation may be at relatively low risk for dementia during their fourth and fifth decades.

As described above, Percy and colleagues[16] noted effects of the ε4 and ε2 alleles on apparent hypothyroidism in older women with DS, but not in men of similar age with DS. Because ε4 is a risk factor for AD in the general population and possibly also for DAD in DS, and ε2 is protective, it was proposed that hypothyroidism may be contributing to DAD at least in women with DS. In an 11-year longitudinal study of one woman with DS who developed DAD, Devenny and colleagues[75] highlighted the difficulties in distinguishing clinical manifestations of DAD from those of depression and hypothyroidism.

Association between thyroid autoimmunity and dementia in Alzheimer's disease in the general population and Down syndrome

The possibility that thyroid autoimmunity may be a peripheral marker for AD has been investigated both in the general population and in people with DS. In the general population there is support for an association between thyroid auto-immunity and DAD. However, statistical data on the sensitivity and specificity of thyroid autoimmunity as a marker for AD are unavailable. Data on the relationship between thyroid autoimmunity and DAD in DS are limited.

Thyroid autoimmunity and dementia in Alzheimer's disease in the general population

Ewins and colleagues[35] investigated the prevalence of autoimmune thyroid disease in familial DAD kindreds without intellectual disability in order to determine whether there was any evidence for genetic linkage between the two disorders. The research involved a large retrospective study of 70 affected and unaffected family members from 12 kindreds. Antithyroglobulin and antimicrosomal autoantibody status was determined. The authors found that 41.1% of the family members showed evidence of autoimmune disease, with significant co-segregation between the presence of thyroid autoantibodies and the development of DAD. The study demonstrated a very high prevalence of autoimmune thyroid disease in familial DAD kindreds, and suggested that a gene for the development of autoimmune thyroid disease may be located on chromosome 21 with close proximity to the familial AD gene. The possibility that thyroid autoimmunity might be a marker for DAD was raised.

Support for an association between thyroid autoimmunity and DAD was subsequently provided by Frecker and colleagues,[38] who found an increase in thyroid autoimmunity in familial DAD cases compared with non-familial DAD cases, and by Genovesi and colleagues,[40] who reported significantly higher levels of both antithyroglobulin and antimicrosomal autoantibody in 34 DAD patients (mean age, 65.17 years; range, 58–75 years) compared with 30 non-demented controls. More recently, Kalmijn and colleagues[48] found that having low TSH levels and autoantibodies to thyroid peroxidase was associated with an especially high risk of DAD. Interestingly, Creutzfeldt–Jacob disease, a neurodegenerative disease associated with altered expression of the prion gene on chromosome 20, is also reported to be associated with a high titre of antithyroid antibodies.[200]

Thyroid autoimmunity and dementia in Alzheimer's disease in Down syndrome

Two studies have been reported for the DS population, with conflicting results. Percy and colleagues[15] investigated thyroid autoimmunity in a study of 46 older people with DS and a group of healthy normal individuals without DS, as already described above. In the latter study it was not possible to age- and gender-match individuals with DS and DAD to those without DAD. However, when corrections for age and gender were applied to individuals with or without DS, individuals with DS and dementia were found to have higher antimicrosomal autoantibody titres than controls without DS, and individuals with DS without dementia had significantly higher antithyroglobulin titres than controls without DS. This study therefore found an association between autoimmune thyroiditis in DS adults with dementia, compared with those without. Prasher,[17] in his study of 201 adults with DS, of whom 27 individuals fulfilled the *ICD–10* criteria for DAD,[199] found no association between the presence of thyroid autoimmunity and DAD. The results from these two studies should be compared with caution because of the differences in methodology. In the former study, antibody titres were compared in cases and controls, whereas in the latter study, frequencies of antibody titres that were above the upper limit of normal were compared. Furthermore, one population was from Canada and the other was from the UK.

Screening and management of thyroid disorders

Screening

It is important to screen for thyroid disorder in people with DS over their entire age range. Some children with DS and hypothyroidism may exhibit decreased growth and development. Symptoms such as obesity, reduced muscle tone, delayed deep tendon reflexes, 'puffy' face, dry skin, constipation, cold intolerance, brittle hair and delayed pubertal development also support the diagnosis of thyroid hormone deficiency. Physical examination of the neck is variable, revealing a thyroid gland that may be normal in size, barely palpable or a diffusely enlarged goitre. Many of these symptoms may be difficult to evaluate, especially in infants. The signs and symptoms of hypothyroidism can develop slowly over time, and may be difficult to discriminate from those of DS itself. Due to increased synthesis and release of thyroid hormone, serum T4 and T3 levels rise, leading to low or suppressed serum TSH. In contrast to the symptoms of hypothyroidism, some children with DS and hyperthyroidism may exhibit tachycardia, tremor, nervousness, sweating, heat intolerance, frequent stools, weight loss, goitre and decreased attention span. However, in contrast to the general population, clinical history and examination are known to be unreliable indicators of thyroid dysfunction in DS. Therefore this population should be regularly screened for thyroid abnormalities. The venous blood test for TSH is used as the gold standard. The capillary blood spot on filter paper to test for TSH is a less costly and more convenient alternative. A filter paper T4 test has also been developed, but is not very sensitive.[9,11,137,138]

Guidelines on best practice for screening vary from one country to another, and some countries do not have them.[201] Most guidelines recommend yearly screening for thyroid disease, as the frequency increases with age. In the USA, screening for thyroid disease at birth, at 6 months of age and yearly thereafter with tests for T4 and TSH is the standard of care.[146] In the UK, the Down Syndrome Medical Interest Group (DSMIG) has recommended screening every two years after the first year of life.[145] A survey of current patterns of screening in the UK was published recently. It was concluded that physicians who completed this survey were complying with the recommended guidelines and that 83% of them were using the venous blood TSH test.[147]

Management

Treatments for thyroid disorders are associated with benefits and risks. The benefits include the restoration of thyroid function if this is abnormal. If thyroid function is not kept within the normal range, the therapy can actually induce disease that is opposite in nature. Both thyroid and antithyroid medications can have harmful effects independently of their effects on thyroid function, and they sometimes have adverse side-effects. Overt hypothyroidism and hyperthyroidism and other thyroid disorders in DS should be treated in the same way as they are in the general population.

Hyperthyroidism

This is treated by one of three modalities, namely antithyroid medications, subtotal or total thyroidectomy, or radioactive iodine ablation.[135,137,184] In many cases these treatments can render the patient euthyroid, but they all have potential adverse effects. Drug treatment may not eliminate recurrences. Pregnant women with hyperthyroidism should be treated with drugs or surgery and not with radioactive iodine, as the latter may have adverse effects on the neonate, such as prematurity, intrauterine growth retardation and fetal or neonatal thyrotoxicosis. Antithyroid medications include the thionamide drugs thiamazole and propylthiouracil. Rare side-effects include rash, itching, fever, liver inflammation or white-blood-cell deficiency. When these drugs are discontinued the problem usually recurs. Radioactive iodine treatment for hyperthyroidism can be administered by mouth without the need for hospitalisation. The majority of patients are cured, but they may end up hypothyroid. Surgical removal of all or part of the thyroid gland as warranted is a permanent cure. This is highly suitable for removing nodules, but not for treating Graves' disease, which affects the whole thyroid. With removal of much or all of the gland comes the need for permanent hypothyroid medication. Surgery also carries the risk of injury to the recurrent laryngeal nerve (the nerve to the voice box).

Hypothyroidism

The treatment of choice for hypothyroidism that is due to insufficient thyroid hormone is levothyroxine sodium (thyroxine). This is a synthetic version of T4, which is converted in the body to T3. This is effective in many cases, although some cases do not respond. An alternative to the commonly used pharmaceuticals is Armour thyroid, a pharmaceutical preparation of purified desiccated pork thyroid tissue that contains significant levels of both T3 and T4. It may be useful in patients suffering from disorders of T4 to T3 conversion. However, excessive use of this preparation has been anecdotally reported to trigger autoimmune-type thyroid disorders, and some people have been reported to develop allergies to it.[137,144]

Subclinical hyperthyroidism and hypothyroidism

The question of whether or not subclinical thyroid abnormalities should be treated is currently controversial. It has been argued by many that it is desirable to be able to prevent overt disease by treating abnormalities at a mild stage of development, or to prevent thyroid disorders and irreversible damage by addressing the primary cause.[130,139–143] On the other hand, treatment that is not necessary may actually cause iatrogenic thyroid disease of the opposite type. Moreover, excess thyroid hormone has harmful effects on the skeletal and cardiovascular systems.

Treatment guidelines

May has published the following guidelines for thyroid screening and treatment in DS.[11]

1 Thyroid function in individuals with DS should be tested annually by measuring T4 and T3 uptake, TSH and T3 levels, and the presence of thyroid autoantibodies.
2 If the T4 value is low (corrected for binding with T3 uptake) and is associated with an elevated TSH level, treat with synthetic thyroid hormone, starting at 25 µg per day after a baseline echocardiogram and electrocardiogram have been obtained. If heart disease is present, baseline Holter monitoring should be undertaken. Increase the thyroid hormone dose by 25 µg every 6 weeks or until the TSH level is normal. Monitor cardiac function carefully.
3 If the TSH level is elevated but the 'corrected' T4 value is normal, repeat the thyroid tests every 6 months, as the natural history of thyroid dysfunction in DS is not well understood and there is always a danger of subclinical medication toxicity.
4 If the autoantibody titres are elevated but the TSH level is normal, continue to monitor annually.
5 If the 'corrected' T4 or T3 value is elevated (i.e. hyperthyroidism), obtain a complete blood cell count and begin treatment with Tapazole 10 mg every 12 hours. Monitor the complete blood cell count frequently initially.

Research studies involving oral supplementation with selenium or zinc

In the introductory section of this chapter we explained how body levels of selenium, zinc and iron can affect thyroid function. The importance of selenium for brain function in the general population is increasingly being recognised.[180] The suggestion that selenium might affect brain function in individuals with DS arose from a literature indicating a direct correlation between cognitive function in people with DS and the activity of red-cell glutathione peroxidase, a seleno-cysteine-containing enzyme. Individuals with DS tend to have lower than normal serum levels of zinc and selenium and higher than normal copper levels.[158] These findings have led to the idea that people with DS might benefit from selective mineral supplementation to improve their thyroid function and cognitive status. However, supplementation studies have not considered the fact that such aberrations in metal ion levels are also characteristic of the acute-phase response.[202] This response consists of a group of physiological changes that occur shortly after the onset of an infection or other inflammatory process, including an increase in the blood level of various proteins (especially C-reactive protein), fever and other metabolic changes. Thus in some instances low serum levels of selenium and/or zinc may be physiologically protective. Observations from published studies on selenium and zinc supplementation in DS are summarised below.

Selenium supplementation
Published effects of selenium supplementation in DS include the following:

- increased plasma and erythrocyte selenium concentrations but decreased red-cell glutathione peroxidase activity after selenium supplementation in children. Children were reported to have fewer infections while taking the selenium[149]
- increased serum concentrations of immunoglobulin G2 and G4 after selenium supplementation in children[203]
- increased red-cell glutathione peroxidase activity.[150]

Zinc supplementation: positive reports
These include the following:

- normalisation of thyroid function tests and white blood cell function[160]
- a significant increase in DNA synthesis; normalisation of the lymphocyte response to phytohaemagglutinin (PHA) up to 6 months after the end of zinc treatment, and lowered response to PHA in half of the patients 22 months after therapy[170]
- normalisation of plasmic zinc, thymulin and TSH levels after 4 months of therapy; decreased incidence of infectious diseases and improved school attendance[204]
- improvement in DNA repair after irradiation[155]
- promotion of increased growth in a proportion of treated children[164]
- reduction in FT3 levels in 17 of 523 patients, and improvement in thyroid function in 9 of 52 patients with low zinc levels[165]
- induction of death of immature white blood cells[172]
- reduction in the number of white blood cells undergoing apoptosis[151]
- correction of abnormally high blood TSH levels in children with low blood zinc levels.[205]

Zinc supplementation: negative and/or adverse reports
These include the following:

- no effect on serum immunoglobulin levels or complement or lymphocyte function. Zinc supplementation may have decreased the frequency and/or severity of infection, as a trend towards fewer sick days was noted anecdotally by parents of participants[162]
- of five patients who presented with recurrent infection and low thymulin levels, three had low cellular zinc levels that normalised after zinc treatment. However, low thymulin levels persisted in four of five patients[152]
- lower T4 and higher TSH levels[25]
- adverse effects on cognitive function in people with AD in the general population. Because people with DS are at high risk of developing dementia at an early age, zinc supplementation in DS may also have adverse consequences.[173] Further studies of this topic are possibly warranted.[154]

Iron supplementation
There have been no reports of iron supplementation to improve thyroid function in DS. It should be noted that too much body iron may result in iron deposition and damage in soft tissues, including the thyroid gland. Interestingly, unusually high levels of iron have been described in adults with DS, particularly those with documented DAD.[206]

Summary and discussion

Causes of thyroid dysfunction

Thyroid dysfunction can result from a number of different causes, either individually or in combination. These include iodine deficiency or excess, defects in the structure or function of the thyroid gland, micronutrient imbalances (including iron, selenium and zinc), genetic causes, structural abnormalities in the hypothalamus and/or pituitary that affect the function of the HPT axis, auto-immune disease associated with the production of antibodies to thyroglobulin, thyroid peroxidase and/or thyroid hormone, and thyroiditis. Thyroid dysfunction can occur at any age. If present, it should be corrected as early as possible to prevent irreversible changes. Treatment is especially important in the neonate in order to promote normal development and function of the brain and the rest of the body. Iodine deficiency is an enormous problem globally. Because it is still the main cause of intellectual and developmental disability worldwide, efforts to eliminate this problem need to be escalated.

Is thyroid function really abnormal in Down syndrome?

There is a large body of evidence indicating that hypothyroidism, both subclinical and overt, is increased in frequency in people with DS, including the newborn.[9,25] In support of the hypothesis that such observations are physiologically mean-ingful, there are a number of observations which indicate that thyroid dysfunc-tion in DS has some unique features – for example, the widespread abnormal histopathology of the thyroid gland in DS, and the fact that autoimmune thyroiditis in adults with DS is associated with the HLA DQA 0301 allele. We speculate that because APP is apparently expressed in the thyroid, and because the gene for this protein is present in triplicate in individuals with DS due to trisomy 21, overexpression of APP may well be a fundamental cause of histopathology of the thyroid gland in DS. On the other hand, it has been suggested that thyroid abnormalities may be no more frequent in DS than they are in the general population, and that published reports contain much false-positive data.[19] The putative false-positive data are due to the fact that the reference ranges used for the diagnosis of thyroid dysfunction in DS are derived from measurements for people without DS. More research needs to be done on this topic.

   Reference ranges should be established specifically for people with DS. Long-itudinal studies of thyroid function in individuals with DS, in which each person serves as their own control, should be particularly informative. Furthermore, attention should be paid to age and gender as well as to diurnal and seasonal variation in measures of tests for thyroid function.

The issue of subclinical hypothyroidism

Because the laboratory reference ranges used to interpret tests of thyroid function are too broad, subclinical hypothyroidism is underdiagnosed in the general population. Because laboratory reference ranges for individuals without DS are used to interpret test results for individuals with DS, subclinical hypothyroidism is likely to be overdiagnosed in DS. The issue of whether or not to treat this disorder in the general population or in individuals with DS has not been resolved. On the one hand, adjustment of thyroid hormone status in the case of mild hypothyroidism may be cognitively beneficial for the intellect. On the other hand, long-term use of synthetic thyroid hormone may have adverse effects on the skeletal and cardiovascular systems. New laboratory reference ranges are warranted for the general population as well as for individuals with DS.

Furthermore, well-designed clinical trials are needed to determine the advantages and/or disadvantages of treating very mild abnormalities of thyroid function in the general population and in individuals with DS.

Association between thyroid dysfunction and Alzheimer's disease in the general population

Although there is a strong rationale for the involvement of thyroid dysfunction, especially hypothyroidism, in AD, our review of studies in this area has not revealed consistent trends. A diagnosis of thyroid dysfunction or changes in the results of biochemical tests of thyroid function are not valid ante-mortem measures of DAD, nor do they have any potentially significant value as a diagnostic marker.

The findings of studies of the involvement of thyroid autoimmunity in DAD appear to be more consistent, raising the possibility that the presence of thyroid autoimmunity might be a peripheral measure for AD. However, researchers have not controlled for subject age or gender as variables. Increasing age and being female are risk factors for both thyroid autoimmunity and DAD. It is therefore unlikely that thyroid autoantibody titres can be used as diagnostic markers for AD.

The possibility cannot be excluded that thyroid dysfunction is involved in some cases of dementia and/or DAD. There are a number of different ways in which this could occur. Certainly long-standing hypothyroidism that is not treated can result in irreversible dementia. In any case of DAD, screening for thyroid dysfunction and several other potentially reversible disorders should be undertaken. Thyroid dysfunction in DAD could also be a result of neuropathological changes in the degenerating brain. Decreased levels of CRH and somatostatin are both characteristic of AD. The former change would lead to decreased TSH secretion, and the latter to increased TSH secretion. It has been reported that somatostatin regulates brain $A\beta42$ through modulation of proteolytic degradation.[207] Changes in thyroid status also could be effected by the stress response, which may be altered in AD as in some other psychiatric illnesses. In the stress response, excessive CRH would stimulate TSH secretion and increase levels of free T4. A raised plasma free T4 level with a normal TSH level is a not uncommon finding in psychiatric illnesses.[208,209] In this case, lowered levels of thyroid-hormone-binding proteins are thought to result in the high levels of free T4. Theoretically, thyroid anomalies in DAD in individuals with DS may result in, or be caused by, the excessive oxidative stress that is characteristic of AD.[10,153,166] Both hypothyroidism and hyperthyroidism are reported to lead to oxidative stress,[158,168,210] which consists of an imbalance between oxidative and antioxidative processes in the body which results in oxidative damage to lipids, nucleic acids and proteins. Oxidative stress can cause cell damage either directly or by altering signalling pathways.[156] Other topics of potential relevance to thyroid dysfunction and DAD are folate deficiency and elevated levels of the amino acid homocysteine, both of which are involved in cognitive decline in ageing.[211] Folate deficiency and high levels of homocysteine are also characteristic of dementia.[211–213] Associations between folate deficiency and hypothyroidism[209] as well as high levels of homocysteine and hypothyroidism[214] have been established. (Folate is a generic term for one of the B vitamins (B_9) that occurs in many different chemical forms and is essential for the synthesis of nucleic acids, the production of methionine from homocysteine, haem synthesis and the production of tyrosine from phenylalanine.[215]) Last but not least, the possibility should be considered that some cases of subclinical thyroid disease among people with DAD reflect physiological defence mechanisms. For example, studies in animals as well as studies of cells and tissues in culture have shown that TSH will counteract cell death resulting from apoptosis (programmed cell death).[216]

As in other disciplines, when controversies arise there are always explanations. We suggest that the failure of subsequent studies to confirm the original findings of Heyman and colleagues[45,46] may be a result of inter-centre differences in one or more of the following factors: criteria used to diagnose DAD; study inclusion/exclusion criteria, including gender, age and stage of dementia; ethnic/genetic background of participants; differences in iodine, selenium, zinc and/or iron status; medications being taken by study participants, such as acetylcholinesterase inhibitors, which may affect thyroid function; and changes in the frequency of untreated hypothyroidism since the 1920s. It is known that hypothyroidism can be masked as DAD, and that if this is not treated at an early stage, the effects can become irreversible. Given that the incidence of hypothyroidism due to iodine deficiency has been gradually decreasing since supplementation of salt with iodine became standard practice in the 1920s, that screening and treatment for hypothyroidism have become increasingly effective, with the development of sensitive methods for measuring thyroid hormone levels since the 1970s, and that screening dementia patients for thyroid abnormality is now standard practice, it would not be surprising to find that the frequency of hypothyroidism (particularly irreversible hypothyroidism) has decreased since Heyman and colleagues conducted their studies in the 1980s, and that currently very few cases of DAD are associated with previous or current thyroid dysfunction.

Association between thyroid dysfunction and dementia of Alzheimer's disease in Down syndrome

More studies are required to determine whether or not there is a connection between thyroid dysfunction and DAD in DS. Although some studies have found no association between thyroid dysfunction and DAD in DS,[16] this possibility has not been excluded.[15,16] Such studies are difficult because, in practice, it is not possible to select groups of people with or without clinical manifestations of AD who are closely matched with regard to age.[15] Furthermore, it is important to keep an open mind as to whether there are differences in the causes of thyroid dysfunction in DS in different countries.

In theory, micronutrient deficiencies of iron, selenium and zinc could result in thyroid dysfunction. The role of imbalances of these nutrients in thyroid disease and in dementia requires further research. One concern is that at least in some cases of apparent zinc and selenium deficiency the micronutrient anomalies may reflect a response to inflammation, and attempts to normalise them might be harmful rather than beneficial. Furthermore, studies of selenium supplementation in geographical areas that are selenium deficient have cautioned that such supplementation should only be undertaken after normalisation of iodine intake, due to the likely upregulation of the selenocysteine deiodinases. Because a literature review indicated that specific vitamin and mineral deficiencies were associated with DS,[148] a placebo-controlled double-blind clinical trial is now under way in the UK to study the effects of supplementation with selenium, zinc and vitamins A, C and E, with or without folinic acid, in babies with DS. The trial outcomes are height, weight, general development, speech and health, and various markers in blood. It will be very interesting to see whether such interventions also affect thyroid status and cognitive status, at least in the short term, and protect against cognitive decline in later years. It could be argued that early treatment of thyroid dysfunction protects one's 'cognitive reserve' later in life. The term 'cognitive reserve' is used to reflect the density of synapses in the brain and also the ability of individuals to function normally despite the presence of histopathological brain features of AD.[217,218]

The topic of folate supplementation and its relationship to thyroid function is of particular interest in the DS population as well as in the general population. People with DS have an unusually high rate of metabolism of folate, due at least in part to their having three copies of the cystathionine β-synthase gene.[167,219,220] In a recent study, serum folate levels were reported to be inversely associated with the level of intellectual disability in people with DS.[221] It would be of great interest to determine whether folate supplementation affects not only the level of intellectual disability, but also thyroid function in DS. Because excess folate is neurotoxic when there is a deficiency of vitamin B_{12}, a balanced B vitamin supplement should be considered instead of folate supplementation on its own.

Management of thyroid disorders

Screening for thyroid dysfunction should be performed in all individuals, including those with DS, over their entire age range. Because thyroid disease appears to be unusually common in people with DS, yearly screening is recommended for this population. As in the general population, if dementia is suspected in older individuals with DS, tests for TSH and vitamin B_{12} levels should be performed, together with tests for other conditions that can mask as DAD, to determine whether there is a reversible cause of the dementia.[29,222] Structural neuroimaging with non-contrast computed tomography or magnetic resonance imaging is also recommended. Other testing should be guided by the history and physical examination. Neuropsychological testing can help to determine the extent of cognitive impairment. When screening for a thyroid disorder, the single best test of thyroid dysfunction is plasma TSH. Measurement of T4 and T3 uptake, T3 levels and the presence of thyroid autoantibodies is also recommended.

Individuals with or without dementia who have overtly abnormal TSH levels and abnormal thyroid hormone test results should be treated. Treatment of individuals with subclinical thyroid disease, with or without dementia, is controversial. The importance of conducting well-designed clinical trials to determine whether treatment has a positive outcome in terms of neurocognitive and/or neurobehavioural functions cannot be overemphasised.

Acknowledgement

The authors thank Tom Dearie, of Hexagram Inc., for providing the artwork for Figure 7.1.

References

1 Benda CE (1946) *Mongolism and Cretinism*. Grune & Stratton, New York.

2 Bosch P, Johnston CE and Karol L (2004) Slipped capital femoral epiphysis in patients with Down syndrome. *J Pediatr Orthop*. **24**: 271–7.

3 Bournville (1903) L'idiotie mongolienne. *Prog Med*. **3**: 117.

4 Evenhuis HM (1991) Frequently occurring but little recognized disorders in adults with Down's syndrome. *Ned Tijdschr Geneeskd*. **135**: 1581–4.

5 Gibson PA, Newton RW, Selby K *et al*. (2005) Longitudinal study of thyroid function in Down's syndrome in the first two decades. *Arch Dis Child*. **90**: 574–8.

6 Hestnes A, Stovner LJ, Husoy O *et al*. (1991) Hormonal and biochemical disturbances in Down's syndrome. *J Ment Defic Res*. **35**: 179–93.

7 Kanavin OJ, Aaseth J and Birketvedt GS (2000) Thyroid hypofunction in Down's syndrome: is it related to oxidative stress? *Biol Trace Elem Res*. **78**: 35–42.

8 Leshin L (2005) *The Thyroid and Down Syndrome*. National Down Syndrome Society, London; www.ndss.org/content.cfm?fuseaction=InfoRes.HlthArticle&article=207 (accessed 7 July 2005).

9 Lovering J and Percy M (2006) Down syndrome. In: I Brown and M Percy (eds) *A Comprehensive Guide to Intellectual and Developmental Disabilities*. Paul H Brookes Publishing, Baltimore, MD.

10 Mihailovic D, Tasic-Dimov D, Mijovic Z *et al*. (2003) Nuclear volume and total optical density in Down syndrome. *Anal Quant Cytol Histol*. **25**: 293–6.

11 May PB (1998) Thyroid dysfunction in Down syndrome: interpretation and management of different patterns of laboratory abnormalities. *Dev Med Rev Rep*. **1(2)**: October. www.altonweb.com/cs/downsyndrome/index.htm?page=thyroidmay.html

12 May P and Kawanishi H (1996) Chronic hepatitis B infection and autoimmune thyroiditis in Down syndrome. *J Clin Gastroenterol*. **23**: 181–4.

13 Nicholson LB, Wong FS, Ewins DL *et al*. (1994) Susceptibility to autoimmune thyroiditis in Down's syndrome is associated with the major histocompatibility class II DQA 0301 allele. *Clin Endocrinol (Oxf)*. **41**: 381–3.

14 Noble J (1998) Natural history of Down's syndrome: a brief review for those involved in antenatal screening. *J Med Screen*. **5**: 172–7.

15 Percy M, Dalton AJ, Markovic D *et al*. (1990) Autoimmune thyroiditis associated with mild 'subclinical' hypothyroidism in adults with Down syndrome: a comparison of patients with and without manifestations of Alzheimer disease. *Am J Med Genet*. **36**: 148–54.

16 Percy ME, Potyomkina Z, Dalton AJ *et al*. (2003) Relation between apolipoprotein E genotype, hepatitis B virus status, and thyroid status in a sample of older persons with Down syndrome. *Am J Med Genet*. **120**: 191–8.

17 Prasher VP (1994) Prevalence of thyroid dysfunction and autoimmunity in adults with Down syndrome. *Down Syndr Res Pract*. **2**: 67–70.

18 Prasher VP (1999) Down syndrome and thyroid disorders: a review. *Down Syndr Res Pract*. **6**: 105–10.

19 Prasher VP and Haque MS (2005) The misdiagnosis of thyroid disorders in Down syndrome: time to re-examine the myth? *Am J Ment Retard*. **110**: 23–7.

20 Rooney S and Walsh E (1997) Prevalence of abnormal thyroid function tests in a Down's syndrome population. *Ir J Med Sci*. **166**: 80–2.

21 Satge D, Ott G, Sasco AJ *et al*. (2004) A low-grade follicular thyroid carcinoma in a woman with Down syndrome. *Tumori*. **90**: 333–6.

22 Seguin E (1866) Idiocy. In: MK Simpson (ed.) *Idiocy: and its treatment by the physiological method*. William Wood & Co., New York.

23 Leshin L (2005) *The Thyroid and Down Syndrome*. National Down Syndrome Society, London; www.ndss.org/content.cfm?fuseaction=InfoRes.HlthArticle&article=207 (accessed 7 July 2005).

24 Storm W (1996) Statistical correlation between increased TSH and increased gliadin antibodies in Down syndrome. *Eur J Pediatr.* **155**: 426.

25 Sustrova M and Strbak V (1994) Thyroid function and plasma immunoglobulins in subjects with Down's syndrome (DS) during ontogenesis and zinc therapy. *J Endocrinol Invest.* **17**: 385–90.

26 Van Trotsenburg AS, Vulsma T, Van Rozenburg-Marres SL *et al.* (2005) The effect of thyroxine treatment started in the neonatal period on development and growth of two-year-old Down syndrome children: a randomized clinical trial. *J Clin Endocrinol Metab.* **90**: 3304–11.

27 Zung A, Yaron A, Altman Y *et al.* (2005) β-Adrenergic hyperresponsiveness in compensated hypothyroidism associated with Down syndrome. *Pediatr Res.* **58**: 66–70.

28 Adelman AM and Daly MP (2005) Initial evaluation of the patient with suspected dementia. *Am Fam Physician.* **71**: 1745–50.

29 Barrett AM (2005) Is it Alzheimer's disease or something else? Ten disorders that may feature impaired memory and cognition. *Postgrad Med.* **117**: 47–53.

30 Belandia B, Latasa MJ, Villa A *et al.* (1998) Thyroid hormone negatively regulates the transcriptional activity of the beta-amyloid precursor protein gene. *J Biol Chem.* **273**: 366–71.

31 Burmeister LA, Ganguli M, Dodge HH *et al.* (2001) Hypothyroidism and cognition: preliminary evidence for a specific defect in memory. *Thyroid.* **11**: 1177–85.

32 Christie JE, Whalley LJ, Bennie J *et al.* (1987) Characteristic plasma hormone changes in Alzheimer's disease. *Br J Psychiatry.* **150**: 674–81.

33 Dobert N, Hamscho N, Menzel C *et al.* (2003) Subclinical hyperthyroidism in dementia and correlation of the metabolic index in FDG-PET. *Acta Med Austriaca.* **30**: 130–3.

34 Edwards JK, Larson EB, Hughes JP *et al.* (1991) Are there clinical and epidemiological differences between familial and non-familial Alzheimer's disease? *J Am Geriatr Soc.* **39**: 477–83.

35 Ewins DL, Rossor MN, Butler J *et al.* (1991) Association between autoimmune thyroid disease and familial Alzheimer's disease. *Clin Endocrinol (Oxf).* **35**: 93–6.

36 Faldt R, Passant U, Nilsson K *et al.* (1996) Prevalence of thyroid hormone abnormalities in elderly patients with symptoms of organic brain disease. *Aging Clin Exp Res.* **8**: 347–53.

37 Foster HD (1987) Disease family trees: the possible roles of iodine in goitre, cretinism, multiple sclerosis, amyotrophic lateral sclerosis, Alzheimer's and Parkinson's diseases and cancers of the thyroid, nervous system and skin. *Med Hypotheses.* **124**: 249–63.

38 Frecker MF, Pryse-Phillips WEM and Strong HR (1994) Immunological associations in familial and non-familial Alzheimer patients and their families. *Can J Neurol Sci.* **21**: 112–19.

39 Ganguli M, Burmeister LA, Seaberg EC *et al.* (1996) Association between dementia and elevated TSH: a community-based study. *Biol Psychiatry.* **40**: 714–25.

40 Genovesi G, Paolini P, Marcellini L *et al.* (1996) Relationship between autoimmune thyroid disease and Alzheimer's disease. *Panminerva Med.* **38**: 61–3.

41 Graebert KS, Lemansky P, Kehle T *et al.* (1995) Localization and regulated release of Alzheimer amyloid precursor-like protein in thyrocytes. *Lab Invest.* **72**: 513–23.

42 Graebert KS, Popp GM, Kehle T *et al.* (1995) Regulated O-glycosylation of the Alzheimer beta-A4 amyloid precursor protein in thyrocytes. *Eur J Cell Biol.* **66**: 39–46.

43 Hayashi M and Patel AJ (1987) An interaction between thyroid hormone and nerve growth factor in the regulation of choline acetyltransferase activity in neuronal cultures derived from the septal-diagonal band region of the embryonic rat brain. *Brain Res.* **433**: 109–20.

44 Hefti F, Hartikka J and Bolger MB (1986) Effect of thyroid hormone analogs on the activity of cholineacetyltransferase in cultures of dissociated septal cells. *Brain Res.* **375**: 413–16.

45 Heyman A, Wilkinson WE, Hurwitz BJ *et al.* (1983) Alzheimer's disease: genetic aspects and associated clinical disorders. *Ann Neurol.* **14:** 507–15.

46 Heyman A, Wilkinson WE, Stafford JA *et al.* (1984) Alzheimer's disease: a study of epidemiological aspects. *Ann Neurol.* **15:** 335–41.

47 Ichibangase A, Nishikawa M, Iwasaka T *et al.* (1990) Relation between thyroid and cardiac functions and the geriatric rating scale. *Acta Neurol Scand.* **81:** 491–8.

48 Kalmijn S, Mehta KM, Pols HA *et al.* (2000) Subclinical hyperthyroidism and the risk of dementia. The Rotterdam study. *Clin Endocrinol (Oxf).* **53:** 733–7.

49 Kapaki E, Ilias I, Paraskevas GP *et al.* (2003) Thyroid function in patients with Alzheimer's disease treated with cholinesterase inhibitors. *Acta Neurobiol Exp (Warsz).* **63:** 389–92.

50 Katzman R, Aronson M, Fuld P *et al.* (1989) Development of dementing illnesses in an 80-year-old volunteer cohort. *Ann Neurol.* **25:** 317–24.

51 Labudova O, Cairns N, Koeck T *et al.* (1999) Thyroid-stimulating-hormone receptor overexpression in brain of patients with Down syndrome and Alzheimer's disease. *Life Sci.* **64:** 1037–44.

52 Latasa MJ, Belandia B and Pascual A (1998) Thyroid hormones regulate beta-amyloid gene splicing and protein secretion in neuroblastoma cells. *Endocrinology.* **139:** 2692–8.

53 Lawlor BA, Sunderland T, Mellow AM *et al.* (1988) Thyroid disease and dementia of the Alzheimer type. *Am J Psychiatry.* **145:** 533–4.

54 Lishman WA (1988) *Organic Psychiatry. The psychological consequences of cerebral disorder* (3e). Blackwell Scientific Publications, Oxford.

55 Lopez O, Huff FJ, Martinez AJ *et al.* (1989) Prevalence of thyroid abnormalities is not increased in Alzheimer's disease. *Neurobiol Aging.* **10:** 247–51.

56 Lopez OL, Becker JT, Klunk W *et al.* (2000) Research evaluation and diagnosis of possible Alzheimer's disease over the last two decades. II. *Neurology.* **55:** 1863–9.

57 Luo L, Yano N, Mao Q *et al.* (2002) Thyrotropin-releasing hormone (TRH) in the hippocampus of Alzheimer patients. *J Alzheimer Dis.* **4:** 97–103.

58 Molchan SE, Lawlor BA, Hill JL *et al.* (1991) The TRH stimulation test in Alzheimer's disease and major depression: relationship to clinical and CSF measures. *Biol Psychiatry.* **30:** 567–76.

59 Quirin-Stricker C, Nappe YV, Simoni P *et al.* (1994) Trans-activation by thyroid hormone receptors of the 5′ flanking region of the human ChAT gene. *Brain Res Mol Brain Res.* **23:** 253–65.

60 Regelson W and Harkins SW (1997) 'Amyloid is not a tombstone' – a summation. The primary role for cerebrovascular and CSF dynamics as factors in Alzheimer's disease (AD): DMSO, fluorocarbon oxygen carriers, thyroid hormonal and other suggested therapeutic measures. *Ann N Y Acad Sci.* **826:** 348–74.

61 Sampaolo S, Campos-Barros A, Mazziotti G *et al.* (2005) Increased cerebrospinal fluid levels of 3,3′,5′-triiodothyronine in patients with Alzheimer's disease. *J Clin Endocrinol Metab.* **90:** 198–202.

62 Schmitt TL, Steiner E, Klingler P *et al.* (1995) Thyroid epithelial cells produce large amounts of the Alzheimer beta-amyloid precursor protein (APP) and generate potentially amyloidogenic APP fragments. *J Clin Endocrinol Metab.* **80:** 3513–19.

63 Schmitt TL, Steiner E, Klinger P *et al.* (1996) The production of an amyloidogenic metabolite of the Alzheimer amyloid beta precursor protein (APP) in thyroid cells is stimulated by interleukin 1 beta, but inhibited by interferon gamma. *J Clin Endocrinol Metab.* **81:** 1666–9.

64 Small GW, Matsuyama SS, Komanduri R *et al.* (1985) Thyroid disease in patients with dementia of Alzheimer type. *J Am Geriatr Soc.* **33:** 538–9.

65 Spiegel J, Hellwig D, Becker G *et al.* (2004) Progressive dementia caused by Hashimoto's encephalopathy – report of two cases. *Eur J Neurol.* **11:** 67.

66 Stern RA, Davis JD, Rogers BL *et al.* (2004) Preliminary study of the relationship between thyroid status and cognitive and neuropsychiatric functioning in euthyroid patients with Alzheimer dementia. *Cogn Behav Neurol.* **17:** 219–23.

67 Sunderland T, Tariot PN, Mueller EA *et al.* (1985) TRH stimulation test in dementia of the Alzheimer type and elderly controls. *Psychiatry Res.* **16:** 269–75.

68 Sutherland MK, Wong L, Somerville MJ *et al.* (1992) Reduction of thyroid hormone receptor c-ERB A alpha mRNA levels in the hippocampus of Alzheimer as compared to Huntington brain. *Neurobiol Aging.* **13:** 301–12.

69 Tappy L, Randin JP, Schwed P *et al.* (1987) Prevalence of thyroid disorders in psychogeriatric inpatients: a possible relationship of hypothyroidism with neurotic depression but not with dementia. *J Am Geriatr Soc.* **35:** 526–31.

70 Thomas DR, Hailwood R, Harris B *et al.* (1987) Thyroid status in senile dementia of the Alzheimer type (SDAT). *Acta Psychiatr Scand.* **76:** 158–63.

71 Van Osch LA, Hogervorst E, Combrinck M *et al.* (2004) Low thyroid-stimulating hormone as an independent risk factor for Alzheimer disease. *Neurology.* **62:** 1967–71.

72 Villa A, Santiago J, Belandia B *et al.* (2004) A response unit in the first exon of the beta-amyloid precursor protein gene containing thyroid hormone receptor and Sp1 binding sites mediates negative regulation by 3,5,3'-triiodothyronine. *Mol Endocrinol.* **18:** 863–73.

73 Bhaumik S, Collacott RA, Garrick P *et al.* (1991) Effect of thyroid-stimulating hormone on adaptive behaviour in Down syndrome. *J Ment Defic Res.* **35:** 512–20.

74 Devenny DA, Silverman WP, Hill AL *et al.* (1996) Normal ageing in adults with Down's syndrome: a longitudinal study. *J Intellect Disabil Res.* **40:** 208–21.

75 Devenny DA, Wegiel J, Schupf N *et al.* (2005) Dementia of the Alzheimer's type and accelerated aging in Down syndrome. *Sci Aging Knowledge Environ.* April 6:(14).

76 MacKhann G, Drachman D, Folstein M *et al.* (1984) Clinical diagnosis of Alzheimer's disease. Report of the NINCDS–ADRDA work group under the auspices of the Department of Health and Human Services Task Force on Alzheimer's disease. *Neurology.* **34:** 939–44.

77 Yoshimasu F, Kokmen E, Hay ID *et al.* (1991) The association between Alzheimer's disease and thyroid disease in Rochester, Minnesota. *Neurology.* **41:** 1745–7.

78 AllThyroid.org (2005) *Your Lifelong Thyroid Resource;* http://AllThyroid.org (accessed 5 July 2005).

79 Andersen S, Bruun NH, Pedersen KM *et al.* (2003) Biologic variation is important for interpretation of thyroid function tests. *Thyroid.* **13:** 1069–78.

80 Andersen S, Pedersen KM, Bruun NH *et al.* (2002) Narrow individual variations in serum T(4) and T(3) in normal subjects: a clue to the understanding of subclinical thyroid disease. *J Clin Endocrinol Metab.* **87:** 1068–72.

81 Borak J (2005) Adequacy of iodine nutrition in the United States. *Conn Med.* **69:** 73–7.

82 Brown R and Larsen PR (2005) *Thyroid Gland Development and Disease in Infants and Children;* www.thyroidmanager.org/Chapter15/15-text.htm (accessed 5 July 2005).

83 Camacho PM and Dwarkanathan AA (1999) Sick euthyroid syndrome. *Postgrad Med Online.* **105:** 215–19.

84 Chanoine JP (2003) Selenium and thyroid function in infants, children and adolescents. *Biofactors.* **19:** 137–43.

85 Cheng SY (2005) Thyroid hormone receptor mutations and disease: beyond thyroid hormone resistance. *Trends Endocrinol Metab.* **16:** 176–82.

86 De Groef B, Vandenborne K, Van As P *et al.* (2005) Hypothalamic control of the thyroidal axis in the chicken: over the boundaries of the classical hormonal axes. *Domest Anim Endocrinol.* **29:** 104–10.

87 De Groot LJ (2004) The non-thyroidal illness syndrome. In: *The Thyroid and its Diseases;* www.thyroidmanager.org/Chapter5/ch5b_text.htm (accessed 7 July 2005).

88 Diagnostic Products Corporation (DPC) (2005) *Thyroid Function. Relationship to other organs;* www.dpcweb.com/medical/thyroid/thyroid_function.html (accessed 5 July 2005).

89 Friesema EC, Jansen J, Milici C *et al.* (2005) Thyroid hormone transporters. *Vitam Horm.* **70:** 137–67.

90 Freake HC, Govoni KE, Guda K *et al.* (2001) Actions and interactions of thyroid hormone and zinc status in growing rats. *J Nutr.* **131:** 1135–41.

91 Harvey CB and Williams GR (2002) Mechanism of thyroid hormone action. *Thyroid.* **12:** 441–6.

92 Kiwanis International (2005) *Serving the Children of the World. Worldwide progress in eliminating iodine deficiency;* www.kiwanis.org/service/wsp/progress.asp (accessed 7 July 2005).

93 Koppe JG (2004) Are maternal thyroid autoantibodies generated by PCBs the missing link to impaired development of the brain? *Environ Health Perspect.* **112:** A862.

94 Kvicala J and Zamrazil V (2003) Effect of iodine and selenium upon thyroid function. *Cent Eur J Public Health.* **11:** 107–13.

95 Laurberg P (2005) Global or Gaelic epidemic of hypothyroidism? *Lancet.* **365:** 738–40.

96 Laurberg P (2005) Towards the global elimination of brain damage due to iodine deficiency: a global program for human development with a model applicable to a variety of health, social and environmental problems. *Thyroid.* **15:** 300.

97 Laurberg P, Bulow Pedersen I, Knudsen N *et al.* (2001) Environmental iodine intake affects the type of nonmalignant thyroid disease. *Thyroid.* **11:** 457–69.

98 Malm J (2004) Thyroid hormone ligands and metabolic diseases. *Curr Pharm Des.* **10:** 3525–32.

99 Michel E, Nauser T, Sutter B *et al.* (2005) Kinetic properties of Cu,Zn-superoxide dismutase as a function of metal content. *Arch Biochem Biophys.* **439:** 234–40.

100 Pimentel L and Hansen KN (2005) Thyroid disease in the emergency department: a clinical and laboratory review. *J Emerg Med.* **28:** 201–9.

101 Refetof S (2001) *Thyroid Hormone Serum Transport Proteins: structure, properties and genes and transcriptional regulation;* www.thyroidmanager.org/Chapter3/3a-frame.htm (accessed 20 October 2005).

102 Rousset BA and Dunn JT (2004) *Thyroid Hormone Synthesis and Secretion;* www.thyroidmanager.org/Chapter2/2-frame.htm (accessed 20 October 2005).

103 Sarne D (2004) Effects of the environment, chemicals and drugs on thyroid function. In: *The Thyroid and its Diseases.* www.thyroidmanager.org/Chapter5/5a-frame.htm (accessed 5 July 2005).

104 Spencer C (2004) *Assay of Thyroid Hormones and Related Substances;* www.thyroidmanager.org/FunctionTests/assay-frame.htm (accessed 20 October 2005).

105 Stockigt J (2004) *Clinical Strategies in the Testing of Thyroid Function;* www.thyroidmanager.org/Chapter6/6b-frame.htm (accessed 5 July 2005).

106 (2005) Thyroid disorders. In: *Merck Manual of Diagnosis and Therapy. Section 2. Endocrine and metabolic disorders;* www.merck.com/mrkshared/mmanual/section2/chapter8/8a.jsp (accessed 20 October 2005).

107 (2005) *Thyroid Disease Manager. The thyroid and its diseases;* www.thyroidmanager.org/thyroidbook.htm (accessed 7 July 2005).

108 (2005) *Thyroid Function Tests. Medical encyclopedia;* www.nlm.nih.gov/medlineplus/ency/article/003444.htm (accessed 7 July 2005).

109 (2005) *Thyroid Hormone Tests. Normal reference ranges;* www.keratin.com/ab/ab011.shtml#03 (accessed 20 October 2005).

110 (2005) *Trace Element and Micronutrient Reference Laboratory;* www.trace-elements.org.uk/bakgrund2.htm (accessed 20 October 2005).

111 Wang HY, Zhang FC, Gao JJ *et al.* (2000) Apolipoprotein E is a genetic risk factor for fetal iodine deficiency disorder in China. *Mol Psychiatry.* **5:** 363–8.

112 Yang J, Feng G, Zhang J *et al.* (2001) Is ApoE gene a risk factor for vascular dementia in Han Chinese? *Int J Mol Med.* **7:** 217–19.

113 Yen PM (2003) Cellular action of thyroid hormone. In: *The Thyroid and its Diseases. Thyroid disease manager;* www.thyroidmanager.org/Chapter3/3d-frame.htm (accessed 7 July 2005).

114 Zetterberg H, Palmer M, Ricksten A *et al.* (2002) Influence of the apolipoprotein E epsilon4 allele on human embryonic development. *Neurosci Lett.* **324:** 189–92.

115 Zimmermann MB and Kohrle J (2002) The impact of iron and selenium deficiencies on iodine and thyroid metabolism: biochemistry and relevance to public health. *Thyroid.* **12:** 867–78.

116 Zoeller RT and Rovet J (2004) Timing of thyroid hormone action in the developing brain: clinical observations and experimental findings. *J Neuroendocrinol.* **16:** 809–18.

117 Saller B, Broda N, Heydarian R *et al.* (1998) Utility of third-generation thyrotropin assays in thyroid function testing. *Exp Clin Endocrinol Diabetes.* **106 (Suppl. 4):** S29–33.

118 Bulow Pedersen I, Knudsen N, Jorgensen T *et al.* (2002) Large differences in incidences of overt hyper- and hypothyroidism associated with a small difference in iodine intake: a prospective comparative register-based population survey. *J Clin Endocrinol Metab.* **87:** 4462–9.

119 Down JLH (1866) Observations on an ethnic classification of idiots. *Clin Lect Rep Med Surg Staff Lond Hosp.* **3:** 259–62.

120 (2005) *Genetics Home References. Congenital hypothyroidism;* http://ghr.nlm.nih.gov/condition=congenitalhypothyroidism (accessed 7 July 2005).

121 (2005) *Guidelines for Diagnosis and Management of Thyroid Disease;* www.thyroidmanager.org/guidelines.htm (accessed 7 July 2005).

122 Ladenson PW (2005) *Section 3. Endocrinology. I. Thyroid;* www.acpmedicine.com/sam/abstracts/0301.htm (accessed 7 July 2005).

123 Levy RP (2005) *Hyperthyroidism;* www.5mcc.com/Assets/SUMMARY/TP0453.html (accessed 7 July 2005).

124 Majeroni BA (2005) *Hypothyroidism, adult;* www.5mcc.com/Assets/SUMMARY/TP0468.html (accessed 5 July 2005).

125 Roberts CG and Ladenson PW (2004) Hypothyroidism. *Lancet.* **363:** 793–803.

126 (2005) *Thyroid Diseases. Medline Plus;* www.nlm.nih.gov/medlineplus/thyroiddiseases.html (accessed 5 July 2005).

127 Weetman AP and De Groot LJ (2004) *Autoimmunity to the Thyroid Gland;* www.thyroidmanager.org/Chapter7/7-frame.htm (accessed 7 July 2005).

128 (2005) *Wrong Diagnosis. Statistics about thyroid disorders;* www.wrongdiagnosis.com/t/thyroid/stats.htm (accessed 7 July 2005).

129 Shalitin S and Phillip M (2002) Autoimmune thyroiditis in infants with Down's syndrome. *J Pediatr Endocrinol Metab.* **15:** 649–52.

130 Bono G, Fancellu R, Blandini F *et al.* (2004) Cognitive and affective status in mild hypothyroidism and interactions with ʟ-thyroxine treatment. *Acta Neurol Scand.* **110:** 59–66.

131 Cooper DS (2004) Thyroid disease in the oldest old: the exception to the rule. *JAMA.* **292:** 2651–4.

132 Gussekloo J, van Exel E, de Craen AJ *et al.* (2004) Thyroid status, disability and cognitive function, and survival in old age. *JAMA.* **292:** 2591–9.

133 Surks MI, Ortiz E, Daniels GH *et al.* (2004) Subclinical thyroid disease: scientific review and guidelines for diagnosis and management. *JAMA.* **291:** 228–38.

134 Volpato S, Guralnik JM, Fried LP *et al.* (2002) Serum thyroxine level and cognitive decline in euthyroid older women. *Neurology.* **58:** 1055–61.

135 De Groot LJ (2005) Diagnosis and treatment of Graves' disease. In: *The Thyroid and its Diseases;* www.thyroidmanager.org/Chapter11/11-frame.htm (accessed 7 July 2005).

136 Benvenga S, Cahnmann HJ and Robbins J (1993) Characterization of thyroid hormone binding to apolipoprotein E: localization of the binding site in the exon-3-coded domain. *Endocrinology.* **133:** 1300–5.

137 Drucker DJ (2005) *MyThyroid.com;* http://mythyroid.com/ (accessed 31 May 2005).

138 Franklyn J and Shephard M (2000) *Evaluation of Thyroid Function in Health and Disease;* http://thyroidmanager.org/Chapter6/6-frame.html (accessed 7 July 2005).

139 Gharib H, Tuttle RM, Baskin HJ *et al.* (2005) Subclinical thyroid dysfunction: a joint statement on management from the American Association of Clinical Endocrinologists, the American Thyroid Association, and the Endocrine Society. *J Clin Endocrinol Metab.* **90:** 581–5.

140 Hoogendoorn EH, Den Heijer M, Van Dijk AP *et al.* (2004) Subclinical hyperthyroidism: to treat or not to treat? *Postgrad Med J.* **80:** 394–8.

141 Prinz PN, Scanlan JM, Vitaliano PP *et al.* (1999) Thyroid hormones: positive relationships with cognition in healthy, euthyroid older men. *J Gerontol A Biol Sci Med Sci.* **54:** M111–16.

142 Smith JW, Evans AT, Costall B *et al.* (2002) Thyroid hormones, brain function and cognition: a brief review. *Neurosci Biobehav Rev.* **26:** 45–60.

143 Van Boxtel MP, Menheere PP, Bekers O *et al.* (2004) Thyroid function, depressed mood, and cognitive performance in older individuals: the Maastricht Aging Study. *Psychoneuroendocrinology.* **29:** 891–8.

144 Wiersinga WM (2004) *Adult Hypothyroidism;* www.thyroidmanager.org/Chapter9/9-frame.htm (accessed 7 July 2005).

145 Down's Syndrome Medical Information Services (2005) *Basic Medical Surveillance Essentials for People with Down's Syndrome. Thyroid disorder;* www.dsmig.org.uk/library/articles/guideline-thyroid-6.pdfwebsite (accessed 7 July 2005).

146 National Down Syndrome Society (2005) *Health Care Guidelines for Individuals with Down Syndrome;* www.ndss.org/content.cfm?fuseaction=InfoRes.HlthArticle&article=37 (accessed 7 July 2005).

147 Varadkar S, Bineham G and Lessing D (2003) Thyroid screening in Down's syndrome: current patterns in the UK. *Arch Dis Child.* **88:** 647.

148 Ani C, Grantham-McGregor S and Muller D (2000) Nutritional supplementation in Down syndrome: theoretical considerations and current status. *Dev Med Child Neurol.* **42:** 207–13.

149 Anneren G, Gebre-Medhin M and Gustavson KH (1989) Increased plasma and erythrocyte selenium concentrations but decreased erythrocyte glutathione peroxidase activity after selenium supplementation in children with Down syndrome. *Acta Paediatr Scand.* **78:** 879–84.

150 Antila E, Nordberg UR, Syvaoja EL *et al.* (1990) Selenium therapy in Down syndrome (DS): a theory and a clinical trial. *Adv Exp Med Biol.* **264:** 183–6.

151 Antonucci A, Di Baldassarre A, Di Giacomo F *et al.* (1997) Detection of apoptosis in peripheral blood cells of 31 subjects affected by Down syndrome before and after zinc therapy. *Ultrastruct Pathol.* **21:** 449–52.

152 Brigino EN, Good RA, Koutsonikolis A *et al.* (1996) Normalization of cellular zinc levels in patients with Down's syndrome does not always correct low thymulin levels. *Acta Paediatr.* **85:** 1370–2.

153 Brooksbank BW and Balazs R (1984) Superoxide dismutase, glutathione peroxidase and lipoperoxidation in Down's syndrome fetal brain. *Brain Res.* **318:** 37–44.

154 Bucci I, Napolitano G, Giuliani C *et al.* (2001) Concerns about using Zn supplementation in Down's syndrome (DS) children. *Biol Trace Elem Res.* **82:** 273–5.

155 Chiricolo M, Musa AR, Monti D *et al.* (1993) Enhanced DNA repair in lymphocytes of Down syndrome patients: the influence of zinc nutritional supplementation. *Mutat Res.* **295:** 105–11.

156 Dryden GW, Deaciuc I, Arteel G *et al.* (2005) Clinical implications of oxidative stress and antioxidant therapy. *Curr Gastroenterol Rep.* **7:** 308–16.

157 DSRF (2005) *Vitamins and Minerals for Children with Down's Syndrome. A randomised controlled trial of the effects of antioxidant and folinic acid supplementation on the mental development, growth and health of children with Down's Syndrome;* www.dsrf.co.uk/Medical_Research/antioxidant%20research%20proj.html (accessed 22 June 2005).

158 Duntas LH and Orgiazzi JV (2003) Vitamin E and thyroid disease: a potential link that kindles hope. *Biofactors.* **19:** 131–5.

159 Kadrabova J, Madaric A, Sustrova M *et al.* (1996) Changed serum trace element profile in Down's syndrome. *Biol Trace Elem Res.* **54:** 201–6.

160 Licastro F, Chiricolo M, Mocchegiani E *et al.* (1994) Oral zinc supplementation in Down's syndrome subjects decreased infections and normalized some humoral and cellular immune parameters. *J Intellect Disabil Res.* **38:** 149–62.

161 Liu G, Garrett MR, Men P *et al.* (2005) Nanoparticle and other metal chelation therapeutics in Alzheimer disease. *Biochim Biophys Acta.* **1741:** 246–52.

162 Lockitch G, Puterman M, Godolphin W *et al.* (1989) Infection and immunity in Down syndrome: a trial of long-term low oral doses of zinc. *J Pediatr.* **114:** 781–7.

163 Mogulkoc R, Baltaci AK, Aydin L *et al.* (2005) The effect of thyroxine administration on lipid peroxidation in different tissues of rats with hypothyroidism. *Acta Physiol Hung.* **92:** 39–46.

164 Napolitano G, Palka G, Grimaldi S *et al.* (1990) Growth delay in Down syndrome and zinc sulphate supplementation. *Am J Med Gene Suppl.* **7:** 63–5.

165 Napolitano G, Palka G, Lio S *et al.* (1990) Is zinc deficiency a cause of subclinical hypothyroidism in Down syndrome? *Ann Genet.* **33:** 9–15.

166 Percy ME, Dalton AJ, Markovic VD *et al.* (1990) Red cell superoxide dismutase, glutathione peroxidase and catalase in Down syndrome patients with and without manifestations of Alzheimer disease. *Am J Med Genet.* **35:** 459–67.

167 Regland B and Gottfries CG (1992) Slowed synthesis of DNA and methionine is a pathogenetic mechanism common to dementia in Down's syndrome, AIDS and Alzheimer's disease? *Med Hypotheses.* **38:** 11–19.

168 Resch U, Helsel G, Tatzber F *et al.* (2002) Antioxidant status in thyroid dysfunction. *Clin Chem Lab Med.* **40:** 1132–4.

169 Sinha S (2004) Anti-oxidant gene expression imbalance, aging and Down syndrome. *Life Sci.* **76:** 1407–26.

170 Stabile A, Pesaresi MA, Stabile AM *et al.* (1991) Immunodeficiency and plasma zinc levels in children with Down's syndrome: a long-term follow-up of oral zinc supplementation. *Clin Immunol Immunopathol.* **58:** 207–16.

171 Thiel R and Fowkes SW (2005) Can cognitive deterioration associated with Down syndrome be reduced? *Med Hypotheses.* **64:** 524–32.

172 Trubiani O, Antonucci A, Palka G *et al.* (1996) Programmed cell death of peripheral myeloid precursor cells in Down patients: effect of zinc therapy. *Ultrastruct Pathol.* **20:** 457–62.

173 Zatta P (2000) Zinc may be a double-faced Janus to Down's syndrome patients. *Biol Trace Elem Res.* **73:** 93–4.

174 Cordes J, Cano J and Haupt M (2000) Reversible dementia in hypothyroidism. *Nervenarzt.* **71:** 588–90.

175 Morganti S, Ceresini G, Nonis E *et al.* (2002) Evaluation of thyroid function in outpatients affected by dementia. *J Endocrinol Invest.* **25 (Suppl. 10):** 69–70.

176 Banerjee B and Chaudhury S (2002) Thyroidal regulation of different isoforms of NaK-ATPase in the primary cultures of neurons derived from fetal rat brain. *Life Sci.* **71:** 1643–54.

177 Laurberg P, Andersen S, Bulow Pedersen I *et al.* (2005) Hypothyroidism in the elderly: pathophysiology, diagnosis and treatment. *Drugs Aging.* **22:** 23–38.

178 Thorne SA, Barnes I, Cullinan P *et al.* (1999) Amiodarone-associated thyroid dysfunction. Risk factors in adults with congenital heart disease. *Circulation.* **100:** 149–54.

179 Basaria S and Cooper DS (2005) Amiodarone and the thyroid. *Am J Med.* **118:** 706–14.

180 Schweizer U, Brauer AU, Kohrle J *et al.* (2004) Selenium and brain function: a poorly recognized liaison. *Brain Res Brain Res Rev.* **45:** 164–78.

181 Visser TJ (2003) *Hormone Metabolism;* www.thyroidmanager.org/Chapter3/3c-frame.htm (accessed 7 July 2005).

182 Mariotti S (2002) *Normal Physiology of the Hypothalamic–Pituitary–Thyroidal System and Relation to the Neural System and Other Endocrine Glands;* www.thyroidmanager.org/Chapter4/4-frame.htm (accessed 7 July 2005).

183 Nishi K, Ichihara K, Takeoka K *et al.* (1996) Intra-individual and seasonal variations of thyroid function tests in healthy subjects. *Rinsho Byori.* **44:** 159–62.

184 Reid JR and Wheeler SF (2005) *Hyperthyroidism: diagnosis and treatment;* www.aafp.org/afp/20050815/contents.html (accessed 7 July 2005).

185 Rovet J and Daneman D (2003) Congenital hypothyroidism: a review of current diagnostic and treatment practices in relation to neuropsychologic outcome. *Paediatr Drugs.* **5:** 141–9.

186 Olivieri A, Stazi MA, Mastroiacovo P *et al.* (2002) Study Group for Congenital Hypothyroidism. A population-based study on the frequency of additional congenital malformations in infants with congenital hypothyroidism: data from the Italian Registry for Congenital Hypothyroidism (1991–1998). *J Clin Endocrinol Metab.* **87:** 557–62.

187 Stoll C, Dott B, Alembik Y *et al.* (1999) Congenital anomalies associated with congenital hypothyroidism. *Ann Genet.* **42:** 17–20.

188 *Wikipedia. Ord's thyroiditis;* http://en.wikipedia.org/wiki/Ord%27s_thyroiditis#Ord.27s_Thyroiditis (accessed 22 October 2005).

189 Jacobs PA, Baikie AG, Court Brown WM *et al.* (1959) The somatic chromosomes in mongolism. *Lancet.* **1:** 710.

190 Lejeune J, Turpin R and Gautier M (1959) Chromosomic diagnosis of mongolism. *Arch Fr Pediatr.* **16:** 962–3.

191 Chao T, Wang JR and Hwang B (1997) Congenital hypothyroidism and concomitant anomalies. *J Pediatr Endocrinol Metab.* **10:** 217–21.

192 Jaruratanasirikul S, Patarakijvanich N and Patanapisarnsak C (1998) The association of congenital hypothyroidism and congenital gastrointestinal anomalies in Down's syndrome infants. *J Pediatr Endocrinol Metab.* **11:** 241–6.

193 Davies P (1979) Neurotransmitter-related enzymes in senile dementia of Alzheimer type. *Brain Res.* **171:** 319–27.

194 Gil-Bea FJ, Garcia-Alloza M, Dominguez J *et al.* (2005) Evaluation of cholinergic markers in Alzheimer's disease and in a model of cholinergic deficit. *Neurosci Lett.* **375:** 37–41.

195 Pierotti AR, Harmar AJ, Simpson J *et al.* (1986) High-molecular-weight forms of somatostatin are reduced in Alzheimer's disease and Down's syndrome. *Neurosci Lett.* **63:** 141–6.

196 Saito T, Iwata N, Tsubuki S *et al.* (2005) Somatostatin regulates brain amyloid beta peptide Abeta42 through modulation of proteolytic degradation. *Nat Med.* **11:** 434–9.

197 Yates CM, Ritchie IM and Simpson J (1981) Noradrenaline in Alzheimer's type dementia and Down syndrome. *Lancet.* **2:** 39–40.

198 Reubi JC and Palacios J (1986) Somatostatin and Alzheimer's disease: a hypothesis. *J Neurol.* **233:** 370–2.

199 World Health Organization (1993) *The ICD–10 Classification of Mental and Behavioural Disorders. Diagnostic criteria for research.* World Health Organization, Geneva.

200 Cossu G, Melis M, Molari A *et al.* (2003) Creutzfeldt–Jakob disease associated with high titer of antithyroid autoantibodies: case report and literature review. *Neurol Sci.* **24:** 138–40.

201 Murphy J, Hoey HM, Philip M *et al.* (2005) Guidelines for the medical management of Irish children and adolescents with Down syndrome. *Ir Med J.* **98:** 48–52.

202 Trace Element and Micronutrient Reference Laboratory (2005) Scottish Trace Element and Micronutrient Reference Laboratory. Scotland's specialised laboratory for trace elements and vitamins in health and disease; www.trace-elements.org.uk/function.htm (accessed 25 October 2005).

203 Anneren G, Magnusson CG and Nordvall SL (1990) Increase in serum concentrations of IgG2 and IgG4 by selenium supplementation in children with Down's syndrome. *Arch Dis Child.* **65:** 1353–5.

204 Licastro F, Mocchegiani E, Zannotti M *et al.* (1992) Zinc affects the metabolism of thyroid hormones in children with Down's syndrome: normalization of thyroid-stimulating hormone and reversal of triiodothyronine plasmic levels by dietary zinc supplementation. *Int J Neurosci.* **65:** 259–68.

205 Bucci I, Napolitano G, Giuliani C *et al.* (1999) Zinc sulfate supplementation improves thyroid function in hypozincemic Down children. *Biol Trace Elem Res.* **82:** 273–5.

206 Prasher VP, Gosling P and Blair J (1998) Role of iron in Alzheimer-type dementia in Down syndrome. *Int J Geriatr Psychiatry.* **13:** 818–19.

207 Higuchi M and Saido TC (2005) Somatostatin regulates brain amyloid beta peptide Abeta42 through modulation of proteolytic degradation. *Nat Med.* **11:** 434–9.

208 Chopra IJ, Solomon DH and Huang TS (1990) Serum thyrotropin in hospitalized psychiatric patients: evidence for hyperthyrotropinemia as measured by an ultrasensitive thyrotropin assay. *Metabolism.* **39:** 538–43.

209 Hein MD and Jackson IMD (1990) Review: thyroid function in psychiatric illness. *Gen Hosp Psychiatry.* **12:** 232–44.

210 Oge A, Sozmen E and Karaoglu AO (2004) Effect of thyroid function on LDL oxidation in hypothyroidism and hyperthyroidism. *Endocr Res.* **30:** 481–9.

211 Kado DM, Karlamangla AS, Huang MH *et al.* (2005) Homocysteine versus the vitamins folate, B_6 and B_{12} as predictors of cognitive function and decline in older high-functioning adults: MacArthur Studies of Successful Aging. *Am J Med.* **118:** 161–7.

212 Barbe F, Klein M, Chango A *et al.* (2001) Homocysteine, folate, vitamin B_{12} and transcobalamins in patients undergoing successive hypo- and hyperthyroid states. *J Clin Endocrinol Metab.* **86:** 1845–6.

213 Malouf M, Grimley EJ and Areosa SA (2003) Folic acid with or without vitamin B_{12} for cognition and dementia (Cochrane Review). In: *The Cochrane Library. Issue 4.* Update Software, Oxford.

214 Nedrebo BG, Nygard O, Ueland PM *et al.* (2001) Plasma total homocysteine in hyper- and hypothyroid patients before and during 12 months of treatment. *Clin Chem.* **47:** 1738–41.

215 *Folinic Acid (5-Formyl Tetrahydrofolate): an active form of folate. Nutritional considerations and applications;* www.folates.com/Folinic%20Acid.htm. (accessed 21 October 2005).

216 Feldkamp J, Pascher E, Perniok A *et al.* (1999) Fas-mediated apoptosis is inhibited by TSH and iodine in moderate concentrations in primary human thyrocytes *in vitro.* *Horm Metab Res.* **31:** 355–8.

217 Whalley LJ, Deary IJ, Appleton CL *et al.* (2004) Cognitive reserve and the neurobiology of cognitive aging. *Ageing Res Rev.* **3:** 369–82.

218 Wolf H, Julin P, Gertz HJ *et al.* (2004) Intracranial volume in mild cognitive impairment, Alzheimer's disease and vascular dementia: evidence for brain reserve? *Int J Geriatr Psychiatry.* **19:** 995–1007.

219 Lejeune J (1990) Pathogenesis of mental deficiency in trisomy 21. *Am J Med Genet Suppl.* **7:** 20–30.

220 Pogribna M, Melnyk S, Pogribny I *et al.* (2001) Homocysteine metabolism in children with Down syndrome: *in vitro* modulation. *Am J Hum Genet.* **69:** 88–95.

221 Gueant JL, Anello G, Bosco P *et al.* (2005) Homocysteine and related genetic polymorphisms in Down's syndrome IQ. *J Neurol Neurosurg Psychiatry.* **76:** 706–9.

222 Prasher V, Percy M, Jozsvai E *et al.* (2006) Outline of Alzheimer disease with implications for people with Down syndrome and other types of intellectual disability. In: I Brown and M Percy (eds) *A Comprehensive Guide to Intellectual and Developmental Disabilities.* Paul H Brookes Publishing, Baltimore, MD.

Chapter 8

Neurophysiological changes associated with dementia in Down syndrome

Frank E Visser, Satnam Kunar and Vee P Prasher

Introduction

The neuropathological changes of Alzheimer's disease (AD), principally senile plaques and neurofibrillary tangles, have been well documented in adults with Down syndrome (DS) and dementia in Alzheimer's disease (DAD). General brain atrophy, a reduction in hippocampus volume and enlargement of the lateral ventricles are all changes that are associated with AD both in the general population and in adults with DS. Not surprisingly, therefore, numerous neurophysiological changes in the brain can also be seen in individuals with DAD.

Historically, due to difficulties in making the clinical diagnosis of DAD in older adults with intellectual disability (ID), and due to the poor validity of neuropsychological measures for detecting AD changes in this population, neurophysiological assessments of brain activity have been undertaken to aid the clinical diagnosis of DAD. Standard electroencephalography (EEG) and evoked potentials are the principal neurophysiological measures used. This chapter will review the role of neurophysiological measures to detect AD changes, highlighting its role in adults with DS.

Electroencephalography

General population

Historically, the principal use of EEG has been to detect abnormal discharge activity in the brain. However, researchers have shown that several non-specific findings on EEG testing are commonly observed in the elderly, and that they are not associated with an increased likelihood of underlying epilepsy. For example, Drury and Beydoun[1] found that 26–35% of adults in the general population over the age of 65 years had interictal epileptiform activity detected on an initial routine EEG assessment. This was thought to be due to the increased frequency of extratemporal seizures in the elderly. Furthermore, periodic lateralising epileptiform discharges can be seen in elderly people without any history of seizures,[2] and intermittent focal slowing in the left temporal region in healthy elderly volunteers.[3,4] The majority of the slowing has been demonstrated to be in the theta range.[5]

In young adults, the average alpha frequency is in the range 10–10.5 Hz.[6] A number of studies have looked at the alpha frequency in healthy elderly subjects and found that at the age of 70 years the average frequency was 9.0–9.5 Hz, falling to 8.5–9.0 Hz after the age of 80 years.[7–9] Other non-specific EEG changes that are seen in the elderly include frontal rhythmic delta activity associated with the onset of drowsiness, subclinical rhythmic electrographic discharges and small sharp spikes and wicket spikes.[10,11]

Down syndrome population

A high prevalence of seizures in individuals with intellectual disability (ID), particularly those with DS, is well established.[12,13] McVicker and colleagues found a prevalence rate for epilepsy of 9.4% in a study based on EEG evidence in individuals with DS living in the community. The prevalence rate of epilepsy increased with age, being particularly high (46%) in those aged over 50 years.[14]

A bimodal distribution of onset of seizures in individuals with DS, consisting of a peak incidence during early childhood and again in middle age, has been described by several authors.[15–17] Other researchers have proposed a triphasic distribution consisting of an increased frequency of seizures during infancy, during early adulthood and in individuals aged 50 years or over.[15,18,19]

Möller and colleagues[19] reported the case of a 55-year-old subject with DS who developed progressively frequent myoclonus and generalised myoclonic–tonic seizures at the age of 52 years. EEG recordings led to the classification of primary generalised epileptic myoclonus. The authors went on to suggest that late-onset myoclonic epilepsy in adults with DS (LOMEDS) should be considered as a differential diagnosis for adult-onset myoclonic epilepsies. The authors argued that LOMEDS shared features with Unverricht–Lundborg disease, a disease caused by a mutation on chromosome 21. Therefore the question of whether there is a specific gene abnormality on chromosome 21 associated with myoclonic epilepsy requires further investigation.

It is well established that adults with DS are at high risk of developing DAD at an earlier age than individuals in the general population.[20–22] Senile plaques similar to those described in AD in the general population were first described in individuals with DS in 1929 by Struwe[23] (who mistakenly attributed them to tuberculosis). More recently, prevalence studies of dementia in adults with DS have demonstrated a dramatic age-specific increase in prevalence rates.[20,24,25] A cross-sectional study conducted in Aarhus, Denmark, found 24% with definite dementia and 24% with possible dementia in the total study population aged 50–60 years with DS.[26] Visser[27] reported a prospective study of institutionalised patients with DS, showing deterioration over a four-year period in 32% of those aged 51–55 years and in 45% of those aged 56–60 years. A second report by Visser and colleagues[28] on 307 institutionalised patients with DS found that the prevalence of dementia increased from 11% for those aged 40–49 years to 77% for those aged 60–69 years. Two individuals aged over 70 years had dementia.

Several researchers have demonstrated an association between late-onset seizures and AD in adults with DS.[29–33] Menendez[29] reported that up to 84% of individuals with DS had seizures. Prasher and Corbett[32] found that late-onset seizures in adults with DS were associated with a poor prognosis, indicating an average life expectancy of less than a further two years, and probable death within three years of the onset of seizures.

Several researchers have suggested that there may be an association between the mental deterioration of patients with DS and an abnormal EEG pattern characterised by the absence of or a very slow alpha rhythm.[20,21,29] Visser and colleagues[33] investigated the role of EEG changes in the diagnosis of DAD in patients with DS. They found that the dominant occipital rhythm became slower at the onset of the cognitive deterioration and eventually disappeared. Changes in the frequency of the dominant occipital rhythm could distinguish between DAD and other causes underlying the cognitive decline. Slowing of the dominant occipital rhythm seemed to be related to DAD in individuals with DS, and its frequency decreased at the onset of cognitive deterioration. Other EEG changes that have been reported to be associated with dementia are an increase in power in the delta and theta bands, with a decrease in beta as well as alpha power.[34,35]

The slowing of the alpha component may develop at a considerably earlier age in individuals with DS than in adults in the general population. A reduction to 8 Hz in adults with DS in their thirties has been reported.[36] It has been suggested that EEG slowing in DS can appear before other signs of dementia in individuals with DS, but it can be difficult to differentiate from simple ageing at this stage.[28] A power spectral analysis performed on occipital EEGs recorded from adults with DS and healthy volunteers demonstrated that the frequencies of occipital alpha rhythms from adults with DS showed a significant inverse correlation with chronological age, whereas the controls did not.[37] A further study also found that older individuals with DS with a decreased alpha background had dementia but also fewer visuo-spatial skills, reduced attention span, larger third ventricles and a global decrease in cerebral glucose utilisation with parietal hypometabolism.[38]

Brunovsky and colleagues[39] assessed the degree of cognitive impairment in individuals with DAD from quantitative EEG indicators. They examined 38 unmedicated patients at various stages of DAD. The EEG recordings showed a decrease in alpha coherence and an increase in delta coherence to be significantly correlated with the degree of dementia. Others have also found a strong correlation between EEG changes and the Mini Mental State Examination (MMSE),[40] which suggested that EEG recordings could supplement the clinical examination. Soininen and colleagues[41] confirmed the findings of Brunovsky and colleagues that changes in EEG recordings were significantly related to MMSE scores and cognitive decline. Partanen and colleagues[42] have concluded that abnormalities in the alpha 'eyes closed/eyes open' ratio in EEG assessments can be used to assess cerebral dysfunction in adults with DS.

Overall, the EEG findings suggest that:

1 there is a strong correlation between EEG changes and cognitive decline, especially slowing of the alpha rhythm
2 in healthy adults with DS such changes may already be seen
3 EEG assessments are of greater value if they are undertaken sequentially
4 EEG changes are not diagnostic for DAD.

Auditory evoked potentials

General population

The auditory evoked potential (AEP) (P3 or P300) response is recorded around 300 milliseconds after a stimulus of an infrequent but relevant tone has been presented in a series of frequent 'ignored' tones. The P300 or 'P3b' component is a scalp positivity that is typically maximal at centroparietal midline sites around 300 milliseconds after the stimulus.[43] Although there is no consensus about the precise cognitive processes underlying the P3 component,[44-46] it is clearly sensitive to attentional resource allocation and working memory load. Factors that influence the P300 size include subjective probability, stimulus saliency, attention and inter-stimulus interval, whereas the P300 is relatively independent of the sensory input characteristics.[47,48] One view is that the P300 reflects the updating of working memory.[45] Although the P300 latency is closely related to the complexity of the stimulus evaluation phase, the P300 amplitude is most sensitive to the subjective probability of the target's occurrence, where decreased probability results in larger amplitudes.[49]

Abnormalities in P300 latency and amplitude have been found in several neurological conditions, including schizophrenia, although most research has focused on an association with dementia.[50-53] P300 latency has been found to be abnormal in healthy elderly people and in moderately demented patients.[54] However, some researchers have found no abnormalities in mildly demented patients.[55,56]

Abnormalities of AEP studies indicate that individuals with DAD in the general population typically have longer P300 latencies (by approximately two standard deviations) and a reduced amplitude size compared with age-matched controls.[51,52,57-59] In the study by Squires and colleagues,[57] the sensitivity of P300 latency for dementia was 80%, compared with only 4% for patients with various psychiatric disorders. In another study,[58] abnormal delay of P300 latency was found in most patients with dementia (80%; age-adjusted value 63%), but in a relatively small percentage of patients with depression and schizophrenia (12% and 13%, respectively). These studies demonstrate that a prolonged P300 latency is not specific to dementia and does not contribute to differential diagnostic procedures. However, it is argued that a patient with equivocal dementia who also has an abnormal P300 has a greatly increased likelihood of having a dementing illness[50] (estimated to be as high as 90%).

Goodin and colleagues[59] reported the findings of a study in which they presented subjects with a series of auditory tones and recorded the resulting evoked potentials. A total of 53 individuals were tested, consisting of 27 patients with dementia and 26 patients with normal mental function but with some other neurological disease (e.g. multiple sclerosis). Dementia was diagnosed using the MMSE.[40] Evoked potentials were compared with data previously collected from 40 normal controls aged 15–76 years. The researchers found that impaired mental functioning in dementia was highly correlated with changes in the latency and amplitude of the P300 component of the AEP. The P300 was delayed in patients with dementia compared with controls, and the P300 abnormalities were not due to neurological disease per se but to dementia.[50]

Pfefferbaum and colleagues[60] also investigated the use of P300 latency in the diagnosis of dementia. Four groups were used, namely 46 cognitively impaired patients (of whom 37 were diagnosed as demented using the MMSE), 20 schizophrenic patients, 34 patients with depression and 115 controls. The demented patients, as a group, had significantly prolonged P300 latencies, but less than half of their latencies fell two or more standard deviations beyond norms. Prolonged P300 latency was also found in the schizophrenic and depressed groups. Abnormal morphology and latency of evoked potentials have been described in vascular dementia as well as DAD,[61,62] and also in Huntington's disease[61] and Parkinson's disease.[63] In addition, P300 abnormalities have been found in the early stages of asymptomatic HIV infection, although they were more frequent and more severe in patients with HIV infection and dementia.[64] However, some studies have not found P300 changes in patients with AD,[65] Korsakoff syndrome[53] or mild vascular dementia.[62]

Polich and colleagues[66] investigated AEP changes in 39 patients with dementia, all of whom met *DSM–III* criteria.[67] Categories for dementia were as follows: DAD, 16 patients (mean age 67.9 years); senile dementia, eight patients (mean age 76.1 years); alcoholic dementia, four patients (mean age 74.5 years); multi-infarct dementia, four patients (mean age 0.8 years); other causes of dementia, seven patients (mean age 70.6 years). Tone stimuli were presented to both ears simultaneously and evoked potentials were recorded from standard scalp points. All groups were found to have prolonged P300 latency and reduced amplitude, which suggests that, at least for this particular sample, effects on P300 latency and amplitude are similar across different aetiologies. However, the authors were able to demonstrate that P300 latency became prolonged as cognitive impairment became more pronounced for a variety of dementing illnesses. Furthermore, some studies indicate that P300 in combination with quantified EEG analysis improves the sensitivity and the discrimination power for separating DAD from other dementias.[68,69]

The use of the P300 component to diagnose dementia is controversial. Slaets and Fortgens[70] studied 71 patients with a mental disorder (42 patients with and 29 patients without dementia) and 19 controls of a much younger age range. The dementia group consisted of patients with senile dementia, multi-infarct dementia, dementia associated with alcoholism and dementia with presenile onset. Only two patients had presenile dementia. The P300 latencies differed significantly between controls and patients in the dementia group, indicating an age-related increase. No significant difference between the demented and non-demented groups was found.

Sara and colleagues[71] compared the results of P300 investigations in 24 patients (aged 61–95 years, mean age 78 years) with dementia, diagnosed according to *ICD–10* and *DSM–III* criteria, and 100 healthy controls (aged 17–92 years), of whom 31 individuals were over the age of 60 years. Of the 24 demented patients, four (17%) were unable to perform the task requirements and therefore did not have a P300 measurement. A further five patients (25%) were excluded. All healthy subjects were able to perform the required task, but 40 out of 150 measurements (26%) were rejected because of contamination. P300 latency was compared in the remaining 15 demented patients and 15 age-matched controls using the two-sample *t*-test. Mean P300 latency did not differ significantly between the two groups. Only 13% of patients with dementia fell outside the two standard error band of the regression of P300 latency on age derived from controls. This study did not demonstrate the usefulness of P300 latency in diagnosing dementia.

Ball and colleagues[72] conducted a longitudinal study of P300 latency in 18 patients with probable DAD. An average of 2.7 recordings per patient were obtained over a period of 34 months. An auditory oddball paradigm was used and subjects kept a count of pitch and loudness. It was found that P300 latency increased over time at a much faster rate in probable DAD patients than in normal controls. This has been observed in other studies that have shown increases in

P300 latency with severity of dementia,[73,74] and it suggests that P300 abnormalities are due to neurodegenerative disease rather than to the ageing process.[43]

Down syndrome population

Late cognitive event-related potentials in adults with DS have been proposed as measures of intellectual decline.[75] Several studies have now been published on the use of AEPs in normal adults with DAD, but few studies have investigated the use of AEPs to detect DAD in the DS population. Blackwood and colleagues[76] performed a study designed to assess the usefulness of the auditory P300 response as a measure of the onset of dementia in individuals with DS. AEPs were recorded from 89 individuals with DS, aged 16–66 years. A control group consisting of 29 individuals with ID with fragile X syndrome and 89 normal volunteer controls was also tested. Clinical psychological testing found evidence of dementia in 16 DS subjects but in none of the individuals with fragile X syndrome. There was a marked increase in P300 latency starting at around 37 years of age in the DS population but not in the other two groups. In controls the effect of age on P300 latency became significant about 17 years later, at the age of around 54 years. The premature effect of age on P300 in DS was due to the prolonged P300 latency in the 16 subjects who showed signs of dementia. Confirmation that increases in P300 latency reflect the development of DAD was obtained when 65 subjects with DS were followed up and retested two years after the initial recordings. The number of subjects who showed clinical evidence of DAD had increased by a further 14%. Of the subjects who exhibited clinical deterioration over a period of two years, 75% showed an increase in P300 latency. None of the group with fragile X syndrome who were retested showed a significant change after two years.[77]

It should be noted that evoked potentials are strongly influenced by the experimental conditions, by differences in study populations with regard to age, type of dementia and appropriate controls, and by differences in methodology with regard to eliciting the P300 response.[78] P300 latency can usually be found in cohorts that include subjects with moderately severe dementia, but not in studies that only include mildly demented individuals. It is sensitive to changes in central processing speed and shows little dependence on educational or linguistic background.[43] At present P300 latency cannot be recommended as a test for DAD in adults with DS, although it has recently been suggested that P300 is a reliable instrument for assessment of the cognitive response to cholinesterase inhibitors in patients with dementia.[79]

Visual evoked potentials

General population

Over the last 35 years visual evoked potentials (VEPs) have gained acceptance as a diagnostic tool in neuro-ophthalmology. Stimuli in common use include diffuse flashing light and pattern-reversal stimulation. The latter is often the more sensitive technique for detecting ophthalmic pathology, the flash VEP only being affected by gross disorders of vision. In psychiatry the role of VEPs remains controversial, but it is generally accepted that presenile dementia produces a slowing of most of the components of the flash VEP.[80,81]

Visser and colleagues[80] studied 19 adults from the general population with a diagnosis of presenile or senile dementia, of mean age 71.2 years (range 52–88 years). The diagnosis was made on clinical grounds alone, with no psychological testing or neuropathological confirmation. Evoked potentials were recorded from the scalp to flash stimuli (minimum flash interval of at least 2 seconds, and flash duration of 10 milliseconds), and the results were compared with those for a reference group of healthy individuals. The latencies of the majority of evoked potentials were found to be increased in the demented group.

Laurian and colleagues[82] investigated VEPs in ten individuals with generalised dementia (mean age 83.4 years), seven individuals with DAD (mean age 73.5 years) and five non-demented controls (mean age 73.3 years). For each subject, 128 VEPs to flash stimuli were recorded and their average was determined. Recordings were obtained by means of electrodes attached at the vertex and occiput sites. Significant topographical differences between subjects with DAD and controls were found. The mean readings from the occipital region were similar for the three groups. At the vertex, in contrast, the responses in the DAD group differed considerably from those in the other two groups. The VEPs in the DAD group were either very flat or absent. The significance of this finding was uncertain, but the authors considered that it provided valuable information for the study of brain dysfunction in AD.

Although flash-only VEPs had generally been the norm, pattern-evoked-only VEPs were performed by Visser and colleagues[83] on 42 patients with dementia and compared with the results for 40 patients with non-dementing behavioural disorder (mainly depressives) and 51 healthy elderly patients. All of the subjects with dementia fulfilled the criteria for *DSM–III* Progressive Degenerative Dementia. None of the patients were on medication during the week before the test, and no ophthalmological abnormalities other than corrected refraction anomalies were present. The stimulus used was a pattern-reversal checkerboard with readings obtained for 2 minutes. No statistically significant differences were found between the left and right hemispheres in either group, and no significant difference was found in the numbers of VEP peaks. The parameters that differentiated the dementia group from the other two groups were increased latency of late peaks, decreased amplitude of some early peaks and increased amplitude of some late peaks.

Another study[84] investigated the use of both flash and pattern-reversal VEPs in adults from the general population with dementia. Elderly people in a longitudinal memory and ageing project were classified as healthy or mildly, moderately or severely demented. A total of 40 individuals with mild DAD were compared with 40 age-matched healthy controls. The study indicated that the later pattern-reversal components (after 170 milliseconds) were delayed in the mildly demented group compared with the healthy group. However, the major positive component of the flash showed no significant difference.

Wright and colleagues[85] proposed that flash VEPs may be used in conjunction with pattern-reversal VEPs as a diagnostic marker of primary senile dementia following earlier work by Doggett and colleagues[86] and Harding and colleagues,[87] who demonstrated that in individuals with established dementia, the latency of the major positive component of the pattern-reversal VEP was normal, but it was markedly delayed in the flash VEP.

Wright and colleagues[85] studied a group of 17 subjects with a clinical diagnosis of presenile dementia, together with 17 healthy age-matched controls from the general population. In addition, a further 17 patients who were suffering from forgetfulness, confusion and depression, but who showed no evidence of dementia, were included as a patient control group. The latency of the flash P2 component in the dementia group showed significant delay at the $P < 0.001$ level compared with the two control groups. The VEP latency for the pattern-reversal (P100) component was normal and showed no significant delay in any of the three groups.

Harding and colleagues[88] continued the above study and reported the findings for 20 individuals who had been diagnosed with primary senile dementia compared with 20 subjects with cortical atrophy but no dementia and 60 individuals in a control group. The demented group was further subdivided into 10 individuals with established dementia of approximately 4–10 years' duration, and 10 individuals diagnosed as suffering from presenile dementia (designated DAD and one case of Pick's disease). The criteria for diagnosis of dementia were not stated. No patients with known ophthalmic pathology were included in the study. Medication was being taken by some patients, but was thought to have a negligible effect on the latency of the VEP. The results from the control group demonstrated that there was a gradual increase (of the order of 20 milliseconds) in the latency of the flash P2 component with increasing age. However, the latency of the pattern-reversal VEP remained constant. Nine out of ten individuals (90%) with established dementia had significantly delayed flash (P2) VEPs, and six individuals (83%) for whom a latency difference between the flash and pattern-reversal VEPs was available had values outside the normal range (values greater than two standard deviations above the mean for age-matched controls). Seven individuals (70%) with early dementia had delayed flash (P2) VEPs, and eight (80%) had latency differences greater than normal. No significant difference was found in the pattern-reversal latency for any of the groups. The authors concluded that this unusual combination of delayed flash but normal pattern reversal (P2–P100 latency) could be used as a more specific diagnostic indicator for primary presenile dementia (more so than EEG and computerised tomography), with a sensitivity of 80% and a specificity of 100%.

Confirmation of these findings that in presenile dementia the P2 component of the flash VEP is delayed, while the pattern-reversal P100 component is of normal latency, and the suggestion that this unusual combination of results may represent a specific test for the diagnosis of dementia, was further supported by Wright and colleagues.[89] In their study, 91 patients suffering from forgetfulness, confusion and depression were referred for VEP and EEG investigations. Individuals were subdivided, on the basis of clinical symptoms alone, into a group of 41 subjects with evidence of dementia and a patient control group consisting of 50 individuals with affective disorder. A second control group consisting of 30 healthy volunteers of equivalent age was used. It was found that the delay in the flash P2 component in dementia was highly significant ($P < 0.001$) when compared with both the patient control group and the healthy control group. The pattern-reversal P100 component was of normal latency and no significant difference was found between the three groups.

Orwin and colleagues[90] followed the progressive effects of DAD in a 58-year-old woman over a period of three and a half years, from the development of the earliest symptoms to complete mental incapacity. The pattern-reversal VEP remained normal, but the flash VEP gradually slowed from 129 milliseconds in 1981 to 153 milliseconds in 1984. The severity of the abnormality of the flash VEP thus reflected the severity of the dementia. EEG, computerised tomography and psychometric tests indicated generalised cortical disease. This longitudinal case strongly supported the use of flash and pattern-reversal VEPs in the diagnosis of DAD.

Philpot and colleagues[91] provided further support for the hypothesis that P2–P100 latency on VEP testing could be used to diagnose presenile dementia when they recorded flash and pattern-reversal VEPs in 29 patients who fulfilled NINCDS–ADRDA criteria for probable AD. The results were compared with those obtained for groups of normal elderly subjects (n =13) and patients with mild mental impairment not amounting to dementia (n = 12). None of the patients were taking psychotropic drugs or showed evidence of ophthalmic pathology, and all of them had corrected binocular visual acuity of 6/9 or better. Furthermore, all of the patients received a clinical dementia rating. The VEPs recorded from four subjects with severe dementia were flat and indistinct, and due to poor cooperation with the procedure these individuals were excluded from any further analysis. The significant correlation between severity of dementia and flash P2 and the P2–P100 latency measure was confirmed. The P2 component of the flash VEP was significantly delayed in AD patients aged 74 years or less, and correlated with severity, whereas the P100 component of the pattern-reversal VEP remained relatively unchanged. However, the authors concluded that although P2–P100 latency VEPs had proved to be a valid discriminator between demented and non-demented subjects, the use of P2–P100 latency VEPs was limited to a younger age group (below 75 years) and to patients with at least moderately severe AD.

In 1989, Pollock and colleagues[92] performed a meta-analysis (a procedure that allows the quantitative evaluation of a group of studies designed to address a common theme) on a total of 12 articles published in English on research on VEPs in dementia. Only six articles provided enough data for meta-analysis (three were excluded because they did not provide the data necessary for computation of effect sizes, two were excluded because they overlapped with previously reported data and one was excluded because it was specifically designed to compare subjects with dementia who had delayed-flash VEPs with other groups, which could bias the results). The meta-analysis indicated that flash and pattern-reversal latencies of demented patients are significantly longer than those of controls. The pattern-reversal P100 latency of the average subject with dementia occurred 62.9% later than that of controls, and the flash P100 latency was expected to exceed 83.6% of that of controls. The article concluded that flash and pattern-reversal VEPs could distinguish elderly demented patients from age-matched controls.

Some investigators have found abnormal P300 data in subjects with DAD during visual target detection tasks.[59,93] Indeed, Saitoh and colleagues[93] found reduced visual P300 amplitude in patients with mild DAD, whereas the visual P100, N100 and P200 potentials were normal. Tanaka and colleagues found that visual P300 latency correlated more strongly with performance on a visuo-spatial test (Raven's progressive matrices) than it did with MMSE[74] score. The opposite was found with the auditory P300 latency.[75]

Down syndrome population

To date few studies have been published that specifically investigated the use of VEPs in the DS population as a test for diagnosing DAD. Crapper and colleagues[94] reported on the use of VEPs in one DS subject. Five months before his death, a 54-year-old man with DS underwent repeated VEP assessment on three occasions over a 1-month period. For the evoked potentials, a flash of light was delivered every 3 seconds. Data were collected in groups of 50 light flashes. The Stanford–Binet intelligence quotient was 30 at the age of 40 years, and at the age of 54 years the subject's mental age was 2.4 years as measured by the Vineland Social Maturity Scale.[95] Three years before his death, he began to show strong evidence of AD, including reduced vocabulary and inability to find his way around familiar places. One year later he developed generalised epilepsy. During the last year of his life there was marked deterioration, development of stooped gait, difficulty in dressing and feeding, and the patient became bedridden and developed limb rigidity. He died from pneumonia complicated by congestive heart failure. At post-mortem his brain revealed characteristic changes of AD. The authors found that the voltage amplitude of the late component of the averaged VEPs was severely depressed or absent. They recommended further investigations of VEPs in individuals with DS with AD.

Prasher and colleagues[96] investigated the role of flash (P2) VEPs and pattern-reversal (P100) VEPs in detecting DAD in adults with DS. Good-quality recordings were available for 19 subjects. In total, 12 individuals had normal VEP results and no clinical dementia, five had abnormal VEP results and DAD, one had a normal VEP result but had DAD, and one had an abnormal VEP recording but was not demented. However, none of the eight individuals with DS and DAD showed the characteristic VEP changes of delayed flash (P2) and normal pattern-reversal (P100) VEP. The authors concluded that VEP measurements are unlikely to be a useful clinical tool in the diagnosis of DAD in adults with DS.

A number of studies have found abnormalities in VEPs in patients with DAD. The unusual combination of delayed flash but normal pattern reversal (P2–P100 latency) is reported to be highly correlated for the general population. For DS subjects with and without DAD, VEP recordings can be abnormal. However, their diagnostic value for the detection of DAD is limited. Several common health disorders in adults with DS can give rise to abnormal VEP findings (e.g. cataracts, keratoconus).

Olfactory event-related potential

Olfactory event-related potential (OERP) may be useful for assessing people with DS who develop dementia. As they show increased dementia, a decrease in olfactory functioning compared with healthy individuals can result. The findings of a study by Wetter and Murphy[97] suggest that the OERP may be a useful measure of olfactory dysfunction in DS, which may precede the development of dementia in these patients.

Conclusion

At present, neurophysiological investigations of DAD in adults with DS have not been fully researched, and are often underused. Specific changes in the EEG are known to occur in people with DS with moderate or severe dementia. These could be used as outcome measures in response to drug treatments where there is uncertainty about the use of standard clinical and neuropsychological measures. The role of evoked potentials is less certain, and further research is required to fully determine their validity in the detection of DAD in people with ID. Serial assessments, with correlation of neurophysiological changes and cognitive decline, would be of particular value. Standard neurophysiological investigations are inexpensive, readily available, can be undertaken on most individuals and can be repeated over time. Their demise is premature.

References

1 Drury I and Beydoun A (1988) Interictal epileptiform activity in elderly patients with epilepsy. *Electroencephalogr Clin Neurophysiol.* **106**: 369–73.
2 Holmes GL (1980) The electroencephalogram as a predictor of seizures following cerebral infarction. *Clin Electroencephalogr.* **11**: 83–6.
3 LaRoche SM and Helmers SL (2003) Epilepsy in the elderly. *Neurologist.* **9**: 241–9.
4 Katz RI and Horowitz GR (1982) Electroencephalogram in the septuagenarian: studies in a normal geriatric population. *J Am Geriatr Soc.* **3**: 273–5.
5 Arenas AM, Brenner RP and Reynolds CF (1986) Temporal slowing in the elderly revisited. *Am J Electroencephalogr Tech.* **26**: 105–14.
6 Brazier MAB and Finesinger JE (1944) Characteristics of the normal encephalogram: a study of the occipital cortical potentials in 500 normal adults. *J Clin Invest.* **23**: 303–6.
7 Otomo E (1966) Electroencephalography in old age: dominant alpha rhythm. *Electroencephalogr Clin Neurophysiol.* **21**: 489–91.
8 Smith MC (1989) Neurophysiology of aging. *Semin Neurol.* **9**: 68–81.
9 Pedley TA and Miller JA (1983) Clinical neurophysiology of aging and dementia. In: R Mayeux and WG Rosen (eds) *The Dementias.* Raven, New York.
10 Katz RI and Horowitz GR (1983) Sleep-onset frontal rhythmic slowing in a normal geriatric population (abstract). *Electroencephalogr Clin Neurophysiol.* **56**: 27.
11 Lee KS and Pedley TA (1997) Electroencephalography and seizures in the elderly. In: AJ Rowan and RE Ramsay (eds) *Seizures and Epilepsy in the Elderly.* Butterworth-Heinemann, Boston, MA.
12 Forsgren L, Edvinsson S-O, Blomquist HK *et al.* (1990) Epilepsy in a population of mentally retarded children and adults. *Epilepsy Res.* **6**: 234–48.
13 Corbett JA (1990) Epilepsy and mental retardation. In: M Dam and L Gram (eds) *Comprehensive Epileptology.* Raven Press, New York.
14 McVicker RW, Shanks OE and McClelland RJ (1994) Prevalence and associated features of epilepsy in adults with Down's syndrome. *Br J Psychiatry.* **164**: 528–32.
15 Pueschel SM, Louis S and McKnight P (1991) Seizure disorders in Down's syndrome. *Arch Neurol.* **48**: 318–20.
16 Prasher VP (1995) Epilepsy and associated effects on adaptive behaviour in Down's syndrome. *Seizure.* **4**: 53–6.
17 Puri BK, Ho KW and Singh I (2001) Age of seizure onset in adults with Down's syndrome. *Int J Clin Pract.* **55**: 442–4.
18 Veall RM (1974) The prevalence of epilepsy among Mongols related to age. *J Ment Defic Res.* **18**: 99–106.
19 Möller JC, Hamer HM, Oertel WH *et al.* (2002) Late-onset myoclonic epilepsy in Down's syndrome (LOMEDS). *Seizure.* **11**: 303–5.
20 Lai F and Williams RS (1989) A prospective study of Alzheimer disease in Down syndrome. *Arch Neurol.* **46**: 849–53.

21 Evenhuis HM (1990) The natural history of dementia in Down's syndrome. *Arch Neurol.* **47**: 263–7.

22 Johanson A, Gustafson J, Brun A *et al.* (1991) A longitudinal study of dementia of Alzheimer type in Down's syndrome. *Dementia.* **2**: 159–68.

23 Struwe F (1929) Histopathologische Untersuchungen über Entstehung und Wesen der senilen Plaques. *Z Gesamte Neurol Psychiatr.* **122**: 291–307.

24 Myers BA and Pueschel SM (1991) Psychiatric disorders in persons with Down syndrome. *J Nerv Ment Dis.* **179**: 609–13.

25 Thase ME, Liss L, Smeltzer D *et al.* (1982) Clinical evaluation of dementia in Down's syndrome: a preliminary report. *J Ment Defic Res.* **26**: 239–44.

26 Johannsen P, Christensen JEJ and Mai J (1996) The prevalence of dementia in Down syndrome. *Dementia.* **7**: 221–5.

27 Visser FE (1993) Clinical diagnosis and prevalence of Alzheimer-type dementia in Down's syndrome. In: MJH Schuurman and DA Flikweet (eds) *Research on Mental Retardation in the Netherlands.* Bishop Bekkers Institute, Utrecht.

28 Visser FE, Aldenkamp AP, Van Huffelen AC *et al.* (1997) Prospective study of the prevalence of Alzheimer-type dementia in institutionalized individuals with Down syndrome. *Am J Ment Retard.* **101**: 400–12.

29 Menendez M (2005) Down syndrome, Alzheimer's disease and seizures. *Brain Dev.* **27**: 246–52.

30 Schrojenstein Lantman-de Valk HMJ, Haveman MJ and Crebolder HFJM (1996) Comorbidity in people with Down's syndrome: a criteria-based analysis. *J Intellect Disabil Res.* **40**: 385–99.

31 Visser FE and Kuilman M (1990) A study of dementia in Down's syndrome of an institutionalized population. *Ned Tijdschr Geneeskd.* **134**: 1141–5.

32 Prasher VP and Corbett JA (1993) Onset of seizures as a poor indicator of longevity in people with Down syndrome and dementia. *Int J Geriatr Psychiatry.* **8**: 923–7.

33 Visser FE, Kuilman M, Oosting J *et al.* (1996) Use of electroencephalography to detect Alzheimer's disease in Down's syndrome. *Acta Neurol Scand.* **94**: 97–103.

34 Angeleri F, Cobianchi A, Giaquinto S *et al.* (1997) Time-series studies: the value of the electroencephalogram in aging, dementia and stroke. In: F Angeleri, S Butler, S Giaquinto and J Majkowski (eds) *Analysis of the Electrical Activity of the Brain.* John Wiley & Sons, Chichester.

35 Schreiter-Gasser U, Gasser T and Ziegler P (1993) Quantitative EEG analysis in early-onset Alzheimer's disease: a controlled study. *Electroencephalogr Clin Neurophysiol.* **86**: 15–22.

36 Katada A, Hasegawa S, Ohira D *et al.* (2000) On chronological changes in the basic EEG rhythm in persons with Down syndrome – with special reference to slowing of alpha waves. *Brain Dev.* **22**: 224–9.

37 Ono Y, Yoshida H, Momotani Y *et al.* (1992) Age-related changes in occipital alpha rhythm of adults with Down syndrome. *Jpn J Psychol Neurol.* **46**: 659–64.

38 Devinsky O, Sato S, Conwit RA *et al.* (1990) Relation of EEG alpha background to cognitive function, brain atrophy and cerebral metabolism in Down's syndrome. Age-specific changes. *Arch Neurol.* **47**: 58–62.

39 Brunovsky M, Matousek M, Edman A *et al.* (2003) Objective assessment of the degree of dementia by means of EEG. *Neuropsychobiology.* **48**: 19–26.

40 Folstein MG, Folstein SE and McHugh PR (1975) Mini-mental state: a practical method for grading the cognitive state of patients for the clinician. *J Psychiatr Res.* **12**: 189–98.

41 Soininen H, Partanen J, Jousmaki V *et al.* (1993) Age-related cognitive decline and electroencephalogram slowing in Down's syndrome as a model of Alzheimer's disease. *Neuroscience.* **53**: 57–63.

42 Partanen J, Soininen H, Kononen M *et al.* (1996) EEG reactivity correlates with neuropsychological test scores in Down's syndrome. *Acta Neurol Scand.* **94**: 242–6.

43 Olichney JM and Hillert DG (2004) Clinical applications of cognitive event-related potentials in Alzheimer's disease. *Phys Med Rehabil Clin North Am.* **15**: 205–33.

44 Picton TW (1992) The P300 wave of the human event-related potential. *J Clin Neurophysiol.* **9**: 456–79.

45 Donchin E (1981) Surprise! . . . Surprise? *Psychophysiology.* **18**: 493–513.

46 Pritchard WS (1981) Psychophysiology of P300. *Psychol Bull.* **89**: 506–40.

47 Johnson R Jr (1986) A triarchic model of P300 amplitude. *Psychophysiology.* **23**: 367–84.

48 Snyder E, Hillyard SA and Galambos R (1980) Similarities and differences among the P3 waves to detected signals in three modalities. *Psychophysiology.* **17**: 112–22.

49 Squires KC, Wickens C, Squires NK *et al.* (1976) The effect of stimulus sequence on the waveform of the cortical event-related potential. *Science.* **193**: 1142–6.

50 Goodin DS, Squires KC and Starr A (1978) Long latency event-related components of the auditory evoked potential in dementia. *Brain.* **4**: 635–48.

51 Brown WS, Marsh JT and La Rue A (1983) Exponential electrophysiological aging: P3 latency. *Electroencephalogr Clin Neurophysiol.* **55**: 277–85.

52 Syndulko K, Hansch EC, Cohen SN *et al.* (1982) Long latency event-related potentials in normal aging and dementia. *Adv Neurol.* **32**: 279–85.

53 St Clair DM, Blackwood DHR and Christie JE (1985) P3 and other long-latency auditory EP in pre-senile dementia, Alzheimer-type and alcoholic Korsakoff syndrome. *Br J Psychiatry.* **147**: 702–6.

54 Polich J (1991) P300 in the evaluation of aging and dementia. In: CHM Brunia, G Mulder G and MN Verbaten (eds) *Event-Related Brain Research.* Elsevier, Amsterdam.

55 Kraiuhin C, Gordon E, Coyle S *et al.* (1990) Normal latency of the P300 event-related potential in mild to moderate Alzheimer's disease and depression. *Biol Psychiatry.* **28**: 372–86.

56 Verleger R, Kömpf D and Neukäter W (1992) Event-related EEG potentials in mild dementia of the Alzheimer type. *Electroencephalogr Clin Neurophysiol.* **84**: 332–43.

57 Squires KC, Chippendale TJ, Wrege KS *et al.* (1980) Electrophysiological assessment of mental functioning in aging and dementia. In: L Poon (ed.) *Aging in the 1980s.* American Psychological Association, Washington, DC.

58 Gordon E, Kraiuhin C, Harris A *et al.* (1986) The differential diagnosis of dementia using P300 latency. *Biol Psychiatry.* **21**: 1123–32.

59 Goodin DS, Squires KC and Starr A (1978) Long latency event-related components of the auditory evoked potential in dementia. *Brain.* **101**: 635–48.

60 Pfefferbaum A, Wenegrat BJ, Ford JM *et al.* (1984) Clinical application of the P3 component of event-related potentials. II. Dementia, depression and schizophrenia. *Electroencephalogr Clin Neurophysiol.* **59**: 104–24.

61 Goodin DS and Aminoff MJ (1986) Electrophysiological differences between subtypes of dementia. *Brain.* **109**: 1103–13.

62 Neshige R, Barrett G and Shibasaki H (1988) Auditory long latency event-related potentials in Alzheimer's disease and multi-infarct dementia. *J Neurol Neurosurg Psychiatry.* **51**: 1120–5.

63 Goodin DS and Aminoff MJ (1987) Electrophysiological differences between demented and non-demented patients with Parkinson's disease. *Ann Neurol.* **21**: 90–4.

64 Goodin DS, Aminoff MJ, Chernoff DN *et al.* (1990) Long latency event-related potentials in patients infected with human immunodeficiency virus. *Ann Neurol.* **27**: 414–19.

65 Knott V, Mohr E, Hache N *et al.* (1999) EEG and the passive P300 in dementia of the Alzheimer type. *Clin Electroencephalogr.* **30**: 64–72.

66 Polich J, Ehlers CL, Otis S *et al.* (1986) P300 latency reflects the degree of cognitive decline in dementing illness. *Electroencephalogr Clin Neurophysiol.* **63**: 138–44.

67 American Psychiatric Association (1987) *Diagnostic and Statistical Manual of Mental Disorders* (revised 3rd edn). American Psychiatric Association, Washington, DC.

68 Jordan S, Nowacki R and Nuwer M (1989) Computerised electroencephalography in the evaluation of early dementia. *Brain Topogr.* **1:** 271–82.

69 Maurer K and Dierks T (1992) Functional imaging procedures in dementias: mapping of EEG and evoked potentials. *Acta Neurol Scand Suppl.* **139:** 40–6.

70 Slaets JPJ and Fortgens C (1984) On the value of P300 event-related potentials in the differential diagnosis of dementia. *Br J Psychiatry.* **45:** 652–6.

71 Sara G, Kraiuhin C, Gordon E *et al.* (1988) The P300 event-related potential component in the diagnosis of dementia. *Aust N Z J Med.* **18:** 657–60.

72 Ball SS, Marsh JT, Schubarth G *et al.* (1989) Longitudinal P300 latency changes in Alzheimer's disease. *J Gerontol A Biol Sci Med Sci.* **44:** 195–200.

73 Patterson JV, Michalewski HJ and Starr A (1988) Latency variability of the components of auditory event-related potentials to infrequent stimuli in aging, Alzheimer-type dementia and depression. *Electroencephalogr Clin Neurophysiol.* **71:** 450–60.

74 Tanaka F, Kachi T, Yamada T *et al.* (1998) Auditory and visual event-related potentials and flash visual evoked potentials in Alzheimer's disease: correlations with Mini-Mental State Examination and Raven's Coloured Progressive Matrices. *J Neurol Sci.* **156:** 83–8.

75 Vieregge P, Verleger R, Schulze-Rava H *et al.* (1992) Late cognitive event-related potentials in adult Down's syndrome. *Biol Psychiatry.* **32:** 1118–34.

76 Blackwood DHR, St Clair DM, Muir WJ *et al.* (1988) The development of Alzheimer's disease in Down's syndrome assessed by auditory event-related potentials. *J Ment Defic Res.* **32:** 439–53.

77 Muir WJ, Squire I, Blackwood DHR *et al.* (1988) Auditory P300 response in the assessment of Alzheimer's disease in Down's syndrome: a 2-year follow-up study. *J Ment Defic Res.* **32:** 455–63.

78 Comi G and Leocani L (2000) Electrophysiological correlates of dementia. *Clin Neurophysiol.* **53:** 331–6.

79 Werber EA, Gandelman-Marton R, Klein C *et al.* (2003) The clinical use of P300 event-related potentials for the evaluation of cholinesterase inhibitor treatment in demented patients. *J Neural Transm.* **110:** 659–69.

80 Visser SL, Stam FC, Van Tilburg W *et al.* (1976) Visual evoked response in senile and presenile dementia. *Electroencephalogr Clin Neurophysiol.* **40:** 385–92.

81 Cosi V, Vitelli E, Gozzoli L *et al.* (1982) Visual evoked potentials in aging of the brain. *Adv Neurol.* **32:** 109–15.

82 Laurian S, Gaillard JM and Wertheimer J (1982) Evoked potentials in the assessment of brain function in senile dementia. In: J Courjon, F Mauguiere and M Revol (eds) *Clinical Applications of Evoked Potentials in Neurology*. Raven Press, New York.

83 Visser SL, Van Tilburg W, Hooijer C *et al.* (1985) Visual evoked potentials (VEPs) in senile dementia (Alzheimer type) and in non-organic behavioural disorders in the elderly: comparison with EEG parameters. *Electroencephalogr Clin Neurophysiol.* **60:** 115–21.

84 Coben LA, Danziger WL and Hughes CP (1983) Visual evoked potentials in mild senile dementia of Alzheimer type. *Electroencephalogr Clin Neurophysiol.* **55:** 121–30.

85 Wright CE, Harding GF and Orwin A (1984) Presenile dementia – the use of the flash and pattern VEP in diagnosis. *Electroencephalogr Clin Neurophysiol.* **57:** 405–15.

86 Doggett CE, Harding GFA and Orwin A (1981) Flash and pattern reversal potentials in patients with presenile dementia (abstract). *Electroencephalogr Clin Neurophysiol.* **52:** 100.

87 Harding GFA, Doggett CE, Orwin A and Smith EJ (1981) Visual evoked potentials in presenile dementia. *Doc Ophthalmol.* **27:** 193–202.

88 Harding GF, Wright CE and Orwin A (1985) Primary presenile dementia: the use of the visual evoked potential as a diagnostic indicator. *Br J Psychiatry.* **147:** 532–9.

89 Wright CE, Harding GFA and Orwin A (1986) The flash and pattern VEP as a diagnostic indicator of dementia. *Doc Ophthalmol.* **62:** 89–96.

90 Orwin A, Wright CE, Harding GF *et al.* (1986) Serial visual evoked potential recordings in Alzheimer's disease. *BMJ.* **293:** 9–10.
91 Philpot MP, Amin D and Levy R (1990) Visual evoked potentials in Alzheimer's disease: correlations with age and severity. *Electroencephalogr Clin Neurophysiol.* **77:** 323–9.
92 Pollock VE, Schneider LS, Chui HC *et al.* (1989) Visual evoked potentials in dementia: a meta-analysis and empirical study of Alzheimer's disease patients. *Biol Psychiatry.* **25:** 1003–13.
93 Saitoh E, Adachi-Usami E, Mizota A *et al.* (2001) Comparison of visual evoked potentials in patients with psychogenic visual disturbance and malingering. *J Pediatr Ophthalmol Strabismus.* **38:** 21–6.
94 Crapper DR, Dalton AJ, Skopitz M *et al.* (1975) Alzheimer degeneration in Down syndrome. Electrophysiological alterations and histopathological findings. *Arch Neurol.* **32:** 618–23.
95 Doll EA (1965) *The Vineland Scale of Social Maturity: condensed manual of directions.* American Guidance Service Inc., Circle Pines, MN.
96 Prasher VP, Krishnan VHR, Clarke DJ *et al.* (1994) Visual evoked potential in the diagnosis of dementia in people with Down syndrome. *Int J Geriatr Psychiatry.* **9:** 473–8.
97 Wetter S and Murphy C (1999) Individuals with Down's syndrome demonstrate abnormal olfactory event-related potentials. *Clin Neurophysiol.* **110:** 1563–9.

Chapter 9

Neuroimaging studies of individuals with Down syndrome

Felix Beacher and Declan G M Murphy

Introduction

In-vivo neuroimaging techniques have several advantages over post-mortem analysis. Most importantly, measurements of brain volume/metabolism are not affected by post-mortem delay or fixation artefacts, and there is also more opportunity to collate cognitive and clinical data on subjects. This chapter will review studies of the brains of individuals with Down syndrome (DS) using five *in-vivo* neuroimaging techniques:

1 single photon emission computed tomography (SPECT)
2 positron emission tomography (PET)
3 proton magnetic resonance spectroscopy (^{1}H-MRS)
4 computerised tomography (CT)
5 magnetic resonance imaging (MRI).

SPECT and PET measure neuronal activity, ^{1}H-MRS measures various aspects of brain metabolism, and CT and MRI can be used to investigate brain anatomy.

SPECT and PET studies of individuals with Down syndrome

SPECT and PET allow *in-vivo* measurement of regional cerebral blood flow (rCBF) and regional glucose consumption, respectively. These are proxy measures of neuronal activity. A number of SPECT and PET studies of individuals with DS have reported abnormalities in rCBF and glucose consumption, both at rest and during performance of cognitive tasks. In addition, SPECT and PET studies of individuals with DS have reported abnormalities in rCBF and glucose metabolism that were related to age and dementia. Abnormalities in rCBF and glucose metabolism are potential confounders for ^{1}H-MRS and volumetric MRI studies of individuals with DS, as abnormalities in rCBF and/or glucose metabolism in individuals with DS may also relate to cognitive deficits and/or dementia. In addition, differences in rCBF and/or glucose metabolism may relate to differences that are detectable using ^{1}H-MRS[1,2] and/or reduced brain volumes, as measured by MRI.[3] SPECT and PET studies of individuals with DS are therefore reviewed here.

SPECT and PET studies of rCBF and glucose metabolism in non-demented individuals with DS

Two SPECT studies have examined rCBF in young, non-demented people with DS.[4,5] Kao and colleagues[4] reported that regional patterns of hypoperfusion (typically unilateral temporal–parietal–occipital deficits) were present in all 14 subjects (age range 8–30 years). Gökçora and colleagues[5] reported that similar patterns of hypoperfusion were present in 8 out of 17 young people with DS (age range 3–24 years), but that the other nine individuals with DS had normal patterns of rCBF. In contrast, one PET study reported that young individuals with DS show no significant differences in glucose consumption compared with healthy controls.[6] The authors therefore suggested that healthy young adults with DS do not show alterations in resting regional brain glucose metabolism which precede neuropathological changes of Alzheimer's disease (AD). Thus there is conflicting evidence that abnormalities in rCBF are present in the brains of younger people with DS even before the development of detectable neurodegenerative changes (for example, as measured by volumetric MRI).

Older, non-demented adults with DS may have age-related abnormalities in rCBF and glucose consumption, as measured by SPECT and PET. One SPECT study of older adults with DS reported that AD-type patterns of rCBF were present in approximately half of the non-demented subjects.[7] The authors suggested that this pattern of hypoperfusion reflects the development of AD neuropathology. Similar results have been reported from PET studies of older, non-demented individuals with DS. For example, one recent PET study reported that both non-demented adults with DS and patients in the general population with dementia in Alzheimer's disease (DAD) had significantly reduced glucose consumption, primarily in the posterior cingulate, compared with age-matched, healthy controls.[8] However, subjects with DS showed significantly *increased* glucose consumption in the inferior temporal/entorhinal cortex compared with healthy controls, whereas individuals with DAD showed significantly *reduced* glucose consumption in these regions compared with healthy controls. These results were replicated after a one-year follow-up. The authors suggested that inferior temporal/entorhinal cortex glucose hypermetabolism in the brains of people with DS may reflect a compensatory response (metabolic 'upregulation') in an early stage of the development of AD. They further suggested that such a compensatory response may subsequently fail, leading to neurodegeneration, glucose hypometabolism and clinically detectable dementia.

In summary, SPECT and PET studies provide some evidence that young individuals with DS may have abnormalities in neuronal metabolism and function that precede the onset of DAD. Furthermore, older non-demented people with DS may have cortical metabolic deficits that are related to the development of 'preclinical' AD-type neuropathology.

PET studies of age-related differences in glucose consumption in non-demented individuals with Down syndrome

Two PET studies have reported that older, non-demented individuals with DS show significant age-related decreases in resting glucose consumption in brain.[9,10]

However, Rondal and Comblain[10] reported that the reduction in resting glucose consumption was not significantly related to differences in measures of cognitive (specifically language) function. The authors thus suggested that an age-related decrease in cortical glucose consumption precedes cognitive decline and/or dementia. In contrast to these studies, two cross-sectional PET studies reported no significant differences in resting glucose metabolism between younger and older non-demented individuals with DS.[11,12] Similarly, a longitudinal PET study of 10 non-demented adults with DS reported that resting brain glucose consumption was stable over an 8- to 12-year period of study.[13] Thus there is mixed evidence as to whether non-demented individuals with DS show significant age-related decreases in resting glucose consumption in brain.

Although there is only limited evidence that non-demented individuals with DS show age-related decreases in *resting* brain glucose consumption, one PET study reported that brain glucose consumption was significantly related to age during cognitive work.[12] This study reported that older individuals with DS had significantly lower rates of glucose consumption in parietal and temporal cortices during an audiovisual stimulation task than younger individuals with DS. The authors interpreted these results as indicating that older people with DS have functional metabolic abnormalities that reflect a 'preclinical' stage of AD.

In summary, some (but not all) PET studies have reported age-related decreases in brain glucose consumption in non-demented individuals with DS. It is proposed that these may be related to the 'preclinical' development of AD.

SPECT and PET studies of individuals with DS and dementia

Both SPECT and PET studies of demented individuals with DS have reported AD-type abnormalities in rCBF and glucose metabolism. For example, SPECT studies have reported that demented people with DS have deficits in rCBF in bilateral temporo-parietal regions, compared with non-demented individuals with DS.[7,14,15] In addition, PET studies have reported that demented individuals with DS have significantly reduced glucose consumption in the parietal and temporal cortices, compared with non-demented DS controls.[16,17] Thus it has been suggested that abnormalities in rCBF and glucose metabolism in individuals with DS and dementia are similar to those in adults from the general population.

Furthermore, one pilot PET study reported that abnormalities in glucose consumption that were able to correctly classify people with and without DAD in the general population were also able to correctly classify all individuals with DS and DAD, and most (88%) of the non-demented DS controls.[18] Another PET study reported that an individual with DS and DAD had significant glucose hypometabolism in the parietal and temporal cortical regions, and at autopsy was found to have a particularly high concentration of AD neuropathology in the same regions.[16] Moreover, a pilot longitudinal PET study reported that two individuals with DS had stable resting brain glucose consumption prior to the onset of dementia, but showed rapid and linear decreases in resting glucose consumption in the temporal and parietal regions following the onset of dementia.[13]

Based on these and other studies it is proposed that:

1 the neuropathology and metabolism of AD is the same in people with DS as it is in the general population

2 AD neuropathology underlies the metabolic abnormalities that are observed in SPECT and PET studies of older people with DS
3 individuals with DS experience a gradual accumulation of AD neuropathology up to a threshold point, after which dramatic changes in brain metabolism occur, associated with clinically detectable dementia.

However, one SPECT study reported that AD abnormalities in rCBF (decreased rCBF in the temporoparietal regions) were present in only one subject out of a sample of five individuals with DS and dementia.[19] This study also reported that similar SPECT abnormalities were present in three out of seven individuals with DS with mild cognitive deterioration, and in 3 out of 14 DS subjects with no cognitive deterioration. Thus the authors found that there was no association between the AD-type SPECT abnormality and either cognitive deterioration or clinical dementia.

In summary, most but not all SPECT and PET studies of individuals with DS and dementia have reported similar patterns of rCBF and glucose metabolism to those that occur in adults in the general population with DAD. This supports the suggestion that there is a similar metabolic process in AD in both populations. However, few studies have directly investigated the potential neural basis for the metabolic abnormalities that are found in individuals with DS and AD.

¹H-MRS studies of individuals with DS

¹H-MRS studies of myo-inositol levels in individuals with DS

Each of the three ¹H-MRS studies of individuals with DS that have measured brain *myo*-inositol levels have reported significant increases in the latter, compared with healthy or learning-disabled control subjects. These increases in *myo*-inositol levels were observed in different brain regions, namely the occipital cortex and parietal white matter,[20] basal ganglia[21] and occipital and parietal regions.[22] It is evident, therefore, that increased *myo*-inositol levels may be widespread in the brain of individuals with DS.

One ¹H-MRS study reported that the *myo*-inositol concentration was increased in two regions of the brain of individuals with DS by approximately 50%, as compared with healthy controls (55% in the occipital cortex and 61% in parietal white matter).[22] The authors proposed that these increases of approximately 50% were due to a proportional gene–dose effect on *myo*-inositol concentration. However, this suggestion is not supported by the other two ¹H-MRS studies of *myo*-inositol in people with DS. These reported a 14% increase in *myo*-inositol/ creatine and phosphocreatine (Cr+PCr)[20] and a 28% increase in *myo*-inositol concentration.[21] One possible explanation for these variations in the magnitude of *myo*-inositol elevation is that they reflect regional variations in *myo*-inositol concentration in the brain. However, other likely sources of variation between these studies include differences in ¹H-MRS protocol and sample composition.

The relationship of myo-inositol concentration in the DS brain to age and dementia

Of the three ¹H-MRS studies of individuals with DS that have measured *myo*-inositol levels, one included only children with DS and did not report age-related differences,[21] and another reported no significant age-related differences in *myo*-inositol levels expressed as a ratio of Cr+PCr.[20] However, one study did describe a significant age-related increase in *myo*-inositol concentration in the occipital lobe.[22] The authors proposed that this age-related increase in *myo*-inositol levels reflected the 'preclinical' development of AD changes in the brains of older individuals with DS, as an increased *myo*-inositol concentration is also observed in AD in adults in the general population.[23] However, this suggestion has not been tested in individuals with DS in the brain regions that are most vulnerable to AD, such as the hippocampus.

Brain *myo*-inositol concentration has only been reported in a single case study of an individual with DS and dementia.[20] No significant further increase in *myo*-inositol concentration was reported in this individual compared with non-demented DS controls. This finding was inconsistent with the numerous reports of an increased brain *myo*-inositol concentration in AD in the general population. However, there are no other ^{1}H-MRS studies of individuals with DS and dementia, and therefore it is not known whether brain *myo*-inositol levels are abnormal in this population.

In summary, the three ^{1}H-MRS studies of subjects with DS that have measured *myo*-inositol levels all reported a significantly increased *myo*-inositol concentration in the brain. Increased *myo*-inositol levels may affect cell function and be related to intellectual disability and/or increased risk of developing DAD in later life. However, no one has related *myo*-inositol concentration to cognitive function or DAD in individuals with DS. The functional significance of abnormal *myo*-inositol levels in the brain of people with DS is therefore unknown.

Other ^{1}H-MRS abnormalities in neuronal integrity in non-demented individuals with DS

Apart from *myo*-inositol, ^{1}H-MRS allows measurement of the levels of other brain metabolites that can be used to assess neuronal integrity. *N*-acetylaspartate (NAA) is a marker of neuronal density[24] and/or mitochondrial function.[25] Choline is a measure of choline-containing compounds, so is used as a measure of membrane turnover.[26] Cr+PCr reflects a cell's phosphate energy metabolism,[24] and is generally stable with respect to disease states and age, so is often used as a reference metabolite. Some studies have therefore expressed the results for ^{1}H-MRS metabolites as ratios of Cr+PCr.

^{1}H-MRS is thus able to measure aspects of neuronal integrity *in vivo*. However, there have been few ^{1}H-MRS studies of neuronal integrity in people with DS, although those that exist have all reported a number of abnormalities in ^{1}H-MRS measures, apart from *myo*-inositol levels.

N-acetylaspartate (NAA) levels in non-demented individuals with DS

One ^{1}H-MRS study of 19 non-demented adults with DS (age range 28–62 years) reported significantly lower NAA levels in both occipital and parietal regions of the DS group, compared with 17 healthy age- and gender-matched controls.[22] However, no significant differences in NAA concentration were reported in three other published ^{1}H-MRS studies of non-demented individuals with DS.[20,21,27] This failure to replicate the finding of decreased NAA levels in people with DS may reflect differences in the samples of DS subjects and control subjects who were studied. For example, Huang and colleagues[22] included only adults with DS, whereas other studies included children with DS.[20, 21] Furthermore, Huang and colleagues[22] compared individuals with DS with healthy controls, whereas Berry and colleagues[21] compared them with non-DS subjects with intellectual disability (ID).

Choline in non-demented individuals with DS

All four published ^{1}H-MRS studies of neuronal integrity in non-demented individuals with DS have reported abnormal levels of choline. However, there are inconsistencies between these three studies.

Three of the four published ^{1}H-MRS studies of neuronal integrity in individuals with DS reported significantly increased levels of choline compared with healthy controls.[20,22,27] However, the magnitude and type of elevation in choline concentration reported by these three studies were dissimilar, being 36% (ratio of choline/Cr+PCr[27]), 11% (choline/Cr+PCr[20]) and 54% and 45% (choline concentration[23]), respectively. Furthermore, one of these studies reported a significantly higher choline/Cr+PCr ratio only in older, not younger, adults with DS, compared with age-matched, healthy controls.[27]

In contrast to these reports of elevated choline levels in people with DS, one ^{1}H-MRS study reported a significantly lower concentration of choline (15% lower) in the basal ganglia of children with DS compared with age-matched controls with ID.[21] However, on balance, ^{1}H-MRS studies may have provided some evidence that choline levels are increased in the brains of adults with DS, compared with healthy controls. It is not yet known whether or how this possible difference in choline levels is related to cognitive function in people with DS.

Creatine and phosphocreatine (Cr+PCr) in non-demented individuals with DS

Of the four ^{1}H-MRS studies of people with DS, only two measured the concentration of Cr+PCr. One of these studies reported no significant differences in Cr+PCr concentration in children with DS, compared with controls with ID.[20] The other study reported a significantly higher concentration of Cr+PCr (9% in occipital and 8% in left parietal region) in non-demented individuals with DS compared with healthy controls.[22] Thus there is some evidence that Cr+PCr levels may be elevated in the brain of adults with DS. However, the significance of a possible increase in Cr+PCr concentration is not known.

Age-related differences in ^{1}H-MRS measures in non-demented individuals with DS

Of the four ^{1}H-MRS studies of non-demented individuals with DS, one did not relate ^{1}H-MRS measures to age,[21] and two found no significant age-related differences in ^{1}H-MRS measures.[20,27] However, significant age-related increases in occipital (but not parietal) *myo*-inositol and Cr+PCr concentrations in non-demented individuals with DS were reported in one study.[22] The healthy control group, by contrast, was reported to show no significant age-related differences in any ^{1}H-MRS measures, and there were significant group x age interactions for *myo*-inositol and Cr+PCr concentration – that is, individuals with DS showed significantly greater age-related increases in these ^{1}H-MRS measures than controls. As noted above, DAD in the general population is also associated with an increase in *myo*-inositol concentration.[23] Thus Huang and colleagues proposed that the increase in *myo*-inositol concentration in older non-demented people with DS reflected the development of 'preclinical' AD in the brain of individuals with DS.[22] However, as already noted, AD-type ^{1}H-MRS differences were not detected by the other two ^{1}H-MRS studies of adults with DS.[20,27] Therefore, taken together, the results of ^{1}H-MRS studies of brain ageing in adults with DS are as yet inconclusive.

A ^{1}H-MRS study of a demented individual with DS

One ^{1}H-MRS study reported significantly lower NAA/Cr+PCr in the occipital cortex and parietal white matter in a single individual with DS and dementia, compared with 23 non-demented DS controls.[20] No significant inter-group differences in other ^{1}H-MRS measures were observed. The authors therefore suggested that a decrease in NAA/Cr+PCr may be an indicator of dementia in people with DS. However, this hypothesis has not been tested in a larger sample of individuals with DS, so to date the ^{1}H-MRS correlates of dementia/AD in people with DS are unknown.

In-vivo neuroimaging studies of brain anatomy in people with DS

There follows a review of studies of brain anatomy in individuals with DS using CT and MRI. Studies using both of these techniques have made significant contributions to our current understanding of brain anatomy in non-demented and demented individuals with DS.

CT studies of brain anatomy in DS

Brain anatomy in non-demented individuals with DS

Brain size is related to head size, so it is important to correct for head size when comparing different groups of people. One CT study of brain anatomy in non-demented individuals with DS reported a number of abnormalities in brain morphology, including significantly smaller corrected volumes of posterior fossa, cerebellum and brainstem, compared with healthy controls.[28] In contrast, another CT study reported that both brain and intracranial volume (i.e. head size) are significantly smaller in people with DS than in healthy controls. However, there was no significant group difference in brain volume after correcting for intracranial volume.[29] In summary, there have been few CT studies comparing brain anatomy in non-demented individuals with DS and in healthy controls. Those that are available offer some evidence of abnormalities in brain anatomy, but these may be partially explained simply by differences in head size.

CT studies relating brain morphology and cognitive function in people with DS

One CT study of a sample that included both non-demented and demented individuals with DS reported that a number of CT measurements (e.g. medial temporal cross-sectional area and lateral ventricle/brain cross-sectional area ratio) were significantly correlated with overall cognitive function as measured by the Mini Mental State Examination (MMSE).[30] However, as this study used a sample which combined both non-demented and demented individuals with DS, the reported correlations may simply reflect the inclusion of subjects with dementia (and thus with low MMSE scores) who also have significantly smaller brain volumes. It is therefore difficult to draw conclusions from this study about how CT measurements are related to cognitive function in either non-demented or demented individuals with DS. Thus the relationship between CT measurements of brain anatomy and cognitive function in adults with DS is poorly understood.

Brain ageing in non-demented adults with DS

CT studies have provided some evidence of accelerated brain ageing in older, non-demented individuals with DS, and suggest that the pattern of brain atrophy in non-demented adults with DS may be similar to that observed in AD in the general population. One study using serial assessment with CT showed that older, non-demented adults with DS had a significantly increased rate of ventricular dilatation compared with younger adults with DS.[17] Another study reported that a sample consisting of demented and non-demented individuals with DS showed significant age-related increases in measures of medial temporal, anterior sub-cortical and caudate atrophy.[30] In contrast, other CT studies found no evidence of accelerated brain ageing in non-demented adults with DS.[29,31,32] In summary, CT studies have provided mixed evidence as to whether non-demented adults with DS show significantly accelerated brain ageing. This inconsistency is likely to be related to discrepancies in sample composition and CT protocol.

CT studies comparing individuals with DS with and without dementia

CT studies comparing individuals with DS with and without dementia have generally reported brain changes which correspond to those observed in people with DAD in the general population. For example, one CT study reported that individuals with DS and dementia show a significantly increased degree of brain atrophy, as indicated by total cerebrospinal fluid and lateral ventricular volumes, compared with non-demented individuals with DS.[17] Similarly, another CT study reported that all six subjects in a sample of adults with DS and dementia showed significant medial temporal atrophy.[32]

One study examined the CT correlates of different stages of AD in adults with DS.[33] The authors reported that early AD was associated with enlargement of the suprasellar cistern (indicating medial temporal atrophy), which was not present in non-demented individuals with DS. Intermediate and advanced DAD were further associated with generalised cortical brain atrophy, particularly in the temporal and frontal regions. In addition, cortical atrophy was reported to be significantly correlated with severity of dementia. Medial temporal and general-ised cortical atrophy, as measured by CT, is found in non-DS subjects with DAD. Thus the results of CT studies of brain anatomy in individuals with DS and dementia are consistent with brain changes reported in adults with DAD in the general population.

CT measurements of the suprasellar cistern ratio (a measure of medial temporal atrophy) have been reported to be able to distinguish dementia status in people with DS with 78% accuracy,[30] consistent with the findings of CT studies of DAD in the general population.[34] Thus CT may have some diagnostic value for detecting dementia in people with DS. However, a recent longitudinal study reported that CT measurements were not able to predict the development of dementia in people with DS.[32] Thus although CT may have some diagnostic value for DAD in individuals with DS, it may not have prognostic value.

In summary, most CT studies that have compared individuals with DS with and without dementia have reported brain differences associated with dementia which correspond to those observed in adults with DAD in the general population. However, CT measurements do not provide a premorbid indicator of those individuals with DS who will go on to develop dementia.

CT has two important disadvantages compared with MRI. First, it uses ionising radiation, which may pose a health risk, and secondly, it is unable to distinguish clearly between white and grey matter in the brain.

Volumetric MRI studies of brain anatomy in individuals with DS

Volumetric MRI studies of brain anatomy in non-demented individuals with DS

In recent years volumetric MRI studies have considerably advanced our understanding of brain anatomy in people with DS. Given that individuals with DS tend to have relatively small stature and small total cranial volumes, most volumetric MRI studies have made statistical adjustments to enable valid comparisons of brain volumes to be made with healthy controls. Corrections have been made on the basis of three different measurements, namely total cranial volume,[35–37] body size[38] or whole brain volume.[39–41]

Volumetric MRI studies have reported that non-demented individuals with DS have abnormalities in a number of corrected regional brain volumes, but especially in the hippocampus and the cerebellum.[39]

Hippocampal volume in non-demented individuals with DS

All volumetric MRI studies of non-demented individuals with DS that measured hippocampal volume have reported significant decreases in corrected volumes compared with healthy controls.[36,38,40–43] Furthermore, this reduction in hippocampal volume has been reported in children as well as adults with DS.[44] Hippocampal hypoplasia in the brain of individuals with DS is therefore most probably present before the onset of neurodegenerative changes associated with the development of AD.

Unfortunately, neither of the volumetric MRI studies of individuals with DS that used control subjects with ID measured hippocampal volume.[45,46] However, reduced hippocampal volume is not a feature of all people with ID. In people with fragile X syndrome[47] and autism,[48] for example, corrected hippocampal volume is reported to be significantly *increased* compared with healthy controls. Thus reduced hippocampal volume in the brain of people with DS does not appear to simply reflect a non-specific effect of ID.

The relationship between putative decreases in hippocampal volume in the brain of people with DS and specific aspects of the cognitive phenotype of DS is unclear. Various lines of evidence point to the involvement of the hippocampus in the healthy brain in episodic memory function.[49] Thus it has been suggested that reduced hippocampal volume in non-demented individuals with DS may explain deficits in memory function.[50] In support of this theory, hippocampal (and also amygdala) volumes were reported to be significantly positively correlated with measures of memory function in a sample of 34 non-demented people with DS.[37] However, this finding has not been replicated by other studies.

In summary, there is strong evidence that hippocampal volume is significantly reduced in the brain of individuals with DS, probably from childhood. There is also preliminary evidence that reduced hippocampal volume may partially explain the memory deficits that are a feature of the cognitive profile of DS.

Cerebellar volume in individuals with DS

With one exception,[36] all volumetric MRI studies that have measured cerebellar volume in people with DS have reported significant reductions in corrected volume compared with healthy controls.[36,37,41,43,45,51] Of all the regional volume reductions that have been reported in the brain of people with DS, volume reductions of the cerebellum may be the most pronounced.[38] In contrast, individuals with Williams' syndrome are reported not to show significant reductions in corrected cerebellar volumes compared with healthy controls.[45] Thus the significant reduction in cerebellar volume in people with DS is unlikely to simply reflect the underlying degree of ID.

Traditionally, the human cerebellum has been associated with motor function. Accordingly, it has been proposed that reduced cerebellar volume in people with DS may underlie the hypotonia and difficulties in motor coordination and speech production which are common features of the disorder.[52] The precise role(s) of the cerebellum in healthy brain function remain controversial. However, recent evidence (for example, from lesion and functional imaging studies) has pointed to its involvement in cognitive and language functions in addition to motor function.[53] Consistent with this, the cerebellum is known to have extensive connections to and from the cerebral cortex, including the frontal and prefrontal regions.[53] Accordingly, studies of healthy brain function have variously implicated the cerebellum in cognitive planning,[54] spatial and general intelligence,[55] judging time intervals and velocities,[56] and word retrieval.[57] Thus it has been proposed that reduced cerebellar volumes in the brain of people with DS may be related to difficulties in higher cognitive functions typical of the disorder (such as syntactic processing[45]), in addition to difficulties in motor function. However, the fact remains that the involvement of cerebellar hypoplasia in cognitive impairment and/or other features of DS has not been experimentally investigated, and is therefore still poorly understood.

Other neuroanatomical abnormalities in non-demented individuals with DS

A number of other neuroanatomical abnormalities have been reported in volumetric MRI studies of non-demented individuals with DS. However, these findings have not been consistently replicated. Two volumetric MRI studies reported that non-demented individuals with DS show significant reductions in corrected volume of whole brain compared with healthy controls.[35,38] Two other studies reported that non-demented individuals with DS show significant reductions in corrected volume of frontal cortex compared with healthy controls.[36,51] It has been suggested that this frontal lobe hypoplasia may play a role in impaired language function in non-demented individuals with DS.[51,58]

Non-demented adults with DS are also reported to show a significant increase in corrected volume of putamen compared with healthy controls.[39] The putamen receives projections predominantly from premotor and motor cortices, and appears to play an important role in motor processing.[59] It has therefore been suggested that preservation of basal ganglia structures in the brain of individuals with DS may underlie the relatively superior performance of people with DS on visual–motor tasks such as the rotor pursuit task.[58]

Volumetric MRI studies of non-demented individuals with DS have also reported smaller corrected volumes of total grey matter, white matter,[35] parietal white matter[38] and left amygdala.[42] In addition, individuals with DS are reported to have a significantly increased corrected volume of the third ventricle and parahippocampal gyrus,[38] lateral ventricles,[42] subcortical and parietal grey matter, and temporal white matter,[41] compared with healthy controls. However, these additional findings have not been replicated, and may simply reflect factors such as inconsistencies in volumetric protocol and sample composition. Therefore it is not yet possible to draw conclusions about their potential significance.

A voxel-based morphometry study of non-demented adults with DS

Voxel-based morphometry (VBM) is an automated technique for examining group differences in whole brain morphology. A recent study used VBM to compare brain anatomy in non-demented adults with DS with that in healthy controls.[43] The authors reported that individuals with DS had significant decreases in grey matter in the cerebellum, cingulate gyrus, left medial frontal lobe, right middle/superior temporal gyrus and the CA2/CA3 region of the left hippocampus, compared with healthy controls. Individuals with DS also showed significant decreases in white matter throughout the inferior brainstem compared with healthy controls. In contrast, individuals with DS were reported to show significant increases in grey matter in a superior/caudal portion of the brainstem and left parahippocampal gyrus compared with healthy controls. Individuals with DS showed significant increases in bilateral white matter in the parahippocampal gyri compared with healthy controls. Furthermore, individuals with DS had significant increases in ventricular cerebrospinal fluid compared with healthy controls. These results are broadly consistent with the findings of previous hand-traced region-of-interest (ROI) studies. For example, the ROI studies also reported that individuals with DS showed volume reductions in the hippocampus, cerebellum and frontal regions[36,51] and increases in parahippocampal formation,[38] compared with healthy controls. VBM is claimed to offer a more fine-tuned approach to the study of differences in regional brain anatomy. However, it is technically more complex than ROI methods and it includes statistical modelling assumptions that may not apply to populations known to have marked abnormalities in brain anatomy. Thus at present it is uncertain whether VBM offers a more accurate description of brain anatomy in DS than ROI techniques.

Studies relating brain anatomy and cognitive function in non-demented individuals with DS

The DS population is associated with a specific cognitive profile, but how this is related to abnormalities in brain anatomy is poorly understood. One way of investigating this issue is by examining the statistical correlations between regional brain volumes and measures of cognitive function. However, to date only three volumetric MRI studies of people with DS have directly compared regional brain volumes with cognitive performance.

One study reported that amygdala and hippocampal volumes were both significantly positively correlated with a number of measures of memory function in 34 non-demented individuals with DS.[37] Memory measures were most strongly associated with volume of the left hippocampus and the right amygdala. These results may support the view that disproportionate deficits in memory function in individuals with DS may be underpinned by reductions in hippocampal volume. However, the methodology of this study was limited in that the authors also reported a significant age-related decrease in corrected hippocampal and amygdala volumes, but did not partial out the effect of age in their statistical analysis. Therefore the significant correlations between hippocampal/amygdala volumes and measures of memory function could simply reflect increasing age. Thus the relationship between hippocampal/amygdala volumes and memory function in people with DS is unclear. Furthermore, this study only measured medial temporal volumes, and therefore potential associations between other regional brain volumes and cognitive function were not examined.

Another MRI study of non-demented individuals with DS reported that a measure of non-verbal intelligence was significantly negatively correlated with volume of parahippocampal gyrus[38] – that is, smaller volumes of parahippocampal gyrus were associated with *higher* non-verbal intelligence in individuals with DS. The biological significance of this surprising finding is not known. The authors suggested that people with DS with larger parahippocampal gyrus volumes may have a more severe form of DS, and may therefore have a more pronounced degree of ID. However, there is no other evidence for this, and this finding has not been replicated by subsequent MRI studies. Therefore this result is difficult to interpret and does not appear to add significantly to our understanding of ID in people with DS.

A recent MRI study of non-demented subjects with DS reported that cross-sectional area of the corpus callosum was significantly positively correlated with overall cognitive function as measured by the Peabody Picture Vocabulary Test, Revised.[60] Corpus callosum atrophy is proposed to be a marker of neocortical atrophy in the AD brain.[61] Teipel and colleagues[62] therefore inferred that callosal atrophy may indicate more general neocortical atrophy in non-demented individuals with DS. VBM analysis of the same data showed significant correlations between memory performance (but not overall cognitive ability) and grey matter volume of the left superior and middle temporal gyrus, bilateral precuneus, left hippocampus, right middle temporal gyrus and right middle frontal gyrus.[63] Thus the biological validity of the reported correlations between overall cognitive function and cross-sectional area of the corpus callosum is probably low.

In summary, to date few MRI studies of non-demented individuals with DS have investigated whether brain anatomy is related to cognitive function. Furthermore, those studies that are available have not added greatly to our understanding of the neurobiological basis of ID in people with DS, either because of methodological limitations or because of difficulties in interpreting results. Therefore the relationship between abnormalities in brain anatomy and ID in people with DS remains poorly understood. So far no studies have investigated whether differences in brain anatomy are related to cognitive function in individuals with DS and dementia.

MRI studies of brain ageing in non-demented individuals with DS

Most volumetric MRI studies of adults with DS have not examined age-related differences in regional brain volume. Those volumetric MRI studies of individuals with DS that have investigated this question provided evidence that non-demented individuals with DS show significant age-related differences in brain morphometry.[36–38,40, 60,62] For example, volumetric MRI studies of non-demented individuals with DS reported significant age-related decreases in volume of the medial temporal regions, including the hippocampi,[36,60] amygdalae and posterior hippocampal gyrus,[37] and also a significant age-related increase in cross-sectional area of the lateral ventricles.[36] Thus some MRI studies of non-demented adults with DS have reported decreases in medial temporal volume, consistent with the findings of studies of brain ageing in the healthy population.

In contrast, two volumetric MRI studies of non-demented adults with DS reported no significant age-related differences in volume of the hippocampi[38,40] and amygdalae.[40] Another MRI study of non-demented adults with DS reported significant (but mild) brain ageing in the cerebellum, the pyramid of the cerebellar vermis and the caudate.[38] The results of this study suggest that individuals with DS may be subject to ageing of brain regions which are not typically affected in brain ageing in the general population.

One important drawback of these studies is that they did not compare the rates of brain ageing in people with DS and healthy controls. Therefore it is not known whether adults with DS have significantly accelerated brain ageing compared with non-DS subjects.

VBM analysis of the cohort of non-demented individuals with DS studied by Teipel and colleagues[60] showed significant age-related decreases in grey matter in bilateral parietal cortex (mainly the precuneus and inferior parietal lobule), bilateral frontal cortex with left-side predominance (mainly the middle frontal gyrus), left occipital cortex (mainly the lingual cortex), right precentral and left postcentral gyrus, left transverse temporal gyrus and right parahippocampal gyrus.[62] Grey matter was reported to be relatively preserved in the cerebellum, the subcortical nuclei, and the basal regions of the frontal and temporal lobe. The authors suggested that this regional pattern of decreases in grey matter was broadly consistent with the findings of previous studies of AD in the general population, and was therefore probably related to the development of 'subclinical' AD in the brain of older people with DS. However, this study reported no significant age-related decreases in the hippocampi or entorhinal cortex, despite the fact that these were previously reported by ROI analysis of the same subjects.[60] The authors concluded that VBM may be less accurate than ROI analysis for certain small brain structures, such as the hippocampus, where there is a close convolution of grey and white matter. It is therefore unclear at present how the results of this VBM study, especially with regard to the hippocampi, relate to previous ROI studies of brain anatomy in the DS population.

In summary, volumetric MRI studies of non-demented adults with DS have provided evidence of significant brain ageing, but have been inconsistent with regard to whether the regional pattern of brain ageing in the DS population is consistent with that typically found in the general population.

Volumetric MRI studies of brain anatomy in demented individuals with DS

Four volumetric MRI studies have examined brain anatomy in individuals with DS and dementia compared with non-demented individuals with DS. However, these studies all used small samples of individuals with DS and dementia (sample size range 2–11), partly due to the practical difficulties of MRI scanning in such a challenging population. However, all four studies provide evidence that individuals with DS and dementia show significant differences in brain anatomy. Furthermore, these studies, although not entirely consistent with each other, are all broadly consistent with volumetric MRI studies of AD in the general population.

Volumetric MRI studies of individuals with DS and dementia have reported a significant reduction in volume of the medial temporal lobe/hippocampus[36,40,42] and neocortex,[36] together with significant enlargement of ventricular CSF.[36,42,63] As already noted, medial temporal and cortical atrophy and ventricular enlargement are neuroanatomical features of AD in the general population. These studies therefore provide evidence that there is most probably a similar pathological process underlying AD in people with DS and in the general population.

However, three of these four MRI studies[36,40,42] used subjects with DS and dementia who were, as a group, significantly older than the non-demented DS controls, but the authors of only one of these studies corrected for subject age in their analysis.[40] As noted above, age is a potentially important confounding factor, because non-demented individuals with DS are reported to show significant age-related differences in regional brain volumes. It is therefore possible that the group differences in regional brain volumes reported by two of the studies[36,42] could simply be explained by the effect of age, rather than by dementia status. However, the authors of one study,[40] which reported that people with DS and dementia had significantly decreased hippocampal volumes, *did* correct for differences in subject age in their analysis. Therefore it is unlikely that volume decreases in the hippocampus in demented individuals with DS can be explained solely by the effect of age.

Of the four MRI studies of demented individuals with DS, only one used an age-matched DS control group.[63] This study reported a trend towards decreased mean hippocampal volumes in individuals with DS, but no significant differences in regional or total brain volume. However, the authors did report that demented individuals with DS had significantly larger total ventricular volumes. Ventricular enlargement is a typical feature of AD in the general population, so the authors concluded that individuals with DS and dementia may undergo changes in brain anatomy that correspond to AD in the general population.

In summary, all four volumetric MRI studies that compared DS subjects with and without dementia have provided evidence for the existence of neuro-anatomical differences in demented DS subjects. Furthermore, these are similar to those reported in AD in the general population. However, there are some inconsistencies between these studies, and some of them did not take into account the confounding effect of age. Thus the neuroanatomical correlates of dementia/AD in people with DS, as measured by MRI, are poorly characterised.

Volumetric MRI studies of non-demented individuals with DS have reported a number of abnormalities in brain anatomy. Most consistently they have reported that individuals with DS have significantly smaller corrected volumes of total brain, cerebellum and hippocampus compared with healthy controls. Significant differences in a number of other regional brain volumes have also been reported, but less consistently. The way in which abnormalities in brain anatomy are related to cognitive function in non-demented DS subjects has been little investigated.

Some MRI studies of brain ageing in non-demented adults with DS have reported significant age-related reductions in volume. However, there are inconsistencies between these studies, and it is not known whether brain ageing in adults with DS is abnormal compared with that in the general population.

Four volumetric MRI studies of individuals with DS with AD/dementia have reported differences in brain anatomy that correspond to those which occur in AD in the general population. However, all of these studies used small samples and most of them suffered from methodological limitations.

Conclusion

Taken together, SPECT and PET studies provide evidence that young people with DS have abnormalities in neuronal metabolism and function which precede the onset of AD. Furthermore, non-demented individuals with DS show age-related differences in brain metabolism which may reflect 'preclinical' accumulation of AD neuropathology, and AD in DS is associated with differences in brain metabolism that are similar to those in the general population. This supports the suggestion that there is a similar metabolic process in AD in both populations.

The four published *in-vivo* ^{1}H-MRS studies of individuals with DS have all reported indications of abnormal neuronal integrity. Their results for NAA, choline and Cr+PCr are somewhat inconsistent. However, the three studies which reported measures of *myo*-inositol all found a significant increase in individuals with DS compared with control subjects. However, the reported magnitude of this elevation in *myo*-inositol concentration has varied considerably. Elevated *myo*-inositol levels in the brain of people with DS may be related both to ID in DS and to increased risk of developing DAD.

Volumetric MRI studies of children and adults with DS have reported a number of abnormalities in brain anatomy. Most consistently, they have reported that non-demented individuals with DS have corrected volume reductions in the cerebellum and hippocampi. Hippocampal hypoplasia may be present from a young age and may be related to deficits in memory function. Cerebellar hypoplasia may be related to deficits in various motor and cognitive functions in individuals with DS. Thus some abnormalities in brain anatomy in DS are relatively well established, but it is unclear how these relate to the cognitive profile of DS. A number of other abnormalities in brain anatomy have also been reported, but less consistently.

In-vivo neuroimaging studies have made significant contributions to our understanding of brain anatomy and metabolism in people with DS, and have reported a number of abnormalities. However, the way in which these abnormalities may be related to cognitive function, age and dementia is still poorly understood.

The role of neuroimaging in the assessment of AD in older adults with DS has not yet been fully evaluated. There are a number of practical issues to be addressed, but if these can be overcome, neuroimaging has a central part to play in our understanding of the biological processes of AD.

References

1 Duncan DB, Herholz K, Kugel H *et al.* (1995) Positron emission tomography and magnetic resonance spectroscopy of cerebral glycolysis in children with congenital lactic acidosis. *Ann Neurol.* **37**: 351–8.

2 Pfund Z, Chugani DC, Juhasz C *et al.* (2000) Evidence for coupling between glucose metabolism and glutamate cycling using FDG PET and ^{1}H magnetic resonance spectroscopy in patients with epilepsy. *J Cereb Blood Flow Metab.* **20**: 871–8.

3 Rostrup E, Knudsen GM, Law I *et al.* (2005) The relationship between cerebral blood flow and volume in humans. *Neuroimage.* **24**: 1–11.

4 Kao CH, Wang PY, Wang SJ *et al.* (1993) Regional cerebral blood flow of Alzheimer's disease-like pattern in young patients with Down's syndrome detected by 99Tcm-HMPAO brain SPECT. *Nucl Med Commun.* **14**: 47–51.

5 Gökçora N, Atasever T, Karabacak NI *et al.* (1999) Tc-99m HMPAO brain perfusion imaging in young Down's syndrome patients. *Brain Dev.* **21**: 107–12.

6 Schapiro MB, Grady CL, Kumar A *et al.* (1990) Regional cerebral glucose metabolism is normal in young adults with Down syndrome. *J Cereb Blood Flow Metab.* **10**: 199–206.

7 Deb S, De Silva PN, Gemmell HG *et al.* (1992) Alzheimer's disease in adults with Down's syndrome: the relationship between regional cerebral blood flow equivalents and dementia. *Acta Psychiatr Scand.* **86**: 340–5.

8 Haier RJ, Alkire MT, White NS *et al.* (2003) Temporal cortex hypermetabolism in Down syndrome prior to the onset of dementia. *Neurology.* **61**: 1673–9.

9 Cutler NR (1986) Cerebral metabolism as measured with positron emission tomography (PET) and [^{18}F] 2-deoxy-D-glucose: healthy aging, Alzheimer's disease and Down syndrome. *Prog Neuropsychopharmacol Biol Psychiatry.* **10**: 309–21.

10 Rondal JA and Comblain A (2002) Language in ageing persons with Down syndrome. *Down Syndr Res Pract.* **8**: 1–9.

11 Schapiro MB, Haxby JV and Grady CL (1992) Nature of mental retardation and dementia in Down syndrome: study with PET, CT and neuropsychology. *Neurobiol Aging.* **13**: 723–34.

12 Pietrini P, Dani A, Furey ML *et al.* (1997) Low glucose metabolism during brain stimulation in older Down's syndrome subjects at risk for Alzheimer's disease prior to dementia. *Am J Psychiatry.* **154**: 1063–9.

13 Dani A, Pietrini P, Furey ML *et al.* (1996) Brain cognition and metabolism in Down syndrome adults in association with development of dementia. *Neuroreport.* **7**: 2933–6.

14 Nakayasu H, Araga S, Takahashi K *et al.* (1991) Two cases of adult Down's syndrome presenting parietal low uptake in ^{123}I-IMP-SPECT. *Rinsho Shinkeigaku.* **31**: 557–60.

15 Puri BK, Zhang Z and Singh I (1994) SPECT in adult mosaic Down's syndrome with early dementia. *Clin Nucl Med.* **19**: 989–91.

16 Schapiro MB, Ball MJ, Grady CL *et al.* (1988) Dementia in Down syndrome: cerebral glucose utilization, neuropsychological assessment and neuropathology. *Neurology.* **38:** 938–42.

17 Schapiro MB, Haxby JV and Grady CL (1992) Nature of mental retardation and dementia in Down syndrome: study with PET, CT and neuropsychology. *Neurobiol Aging.* **13:** 723–34.

18 Azari NP, Horwitz B, Pettigrew KD *et al.* (1994) Abnormal pattern of cerebral glucose metabolic rates involving language areas in young adults with Down syndrome. *Brain Lang.* **46:** 1–20.

19 Jones AM, Kennedy N, Hanson J *et al.* (1997) A study of dementia in adults with Down's syndrome using 99Tc(m)-HMPAO SPECT. *Nucl Med Commun.* **18:** 662–7.

20 Shonk T and Ross BD (1995) Role of increased cerebral myo-inositol in the dementia of DS. *Magn Reson Med.* **33:** 858–61.

21 Berry GT, Wang ZJ, Dreba SF *et al.* (1999). *In vivo* brain myo-inositol levels in children with Down syndrome. *J Pediatr.* **135:** 94–7.

22 Huang W, Alexander GE, Daly EM *et al.* (1999) High brain myo-inositol levels in the predementia phase of Alzheimer's disease in adults with Down's syndrome: a ^{1}H-MRS study. *Am J Psychiatry.* **156:** 1879–86.

23 Firbank MJ, Harrison RM and O'Brien JT (2002) A comprehensive review of proton magnetic resonance spectroscopy studies in dementia and Parkinson's disease. *Dement Geriatr Cogn Disord.* **14:** 64–76.

24 Miller BL (1991) A review of chemical issues in ^{1}H NMR spectroscopy: N-acetyl-L-aspartate, creatine and choline. *NMR Biomed.* **4:** 47–52.

25 Bates T, Strangeward M, Keelan J *et al.* (1996) Inhibition of N-acetylaspartate production: implications for ^{1}H-MRS studies *in vivo. Neuroreport.* **7:** 1397–400.

26 Miller BL, Chang L, Booth R *et al.* (1996) *In vivo* ^{1}H MRS choline: correlation with *in vitro* chemistry/histology. *Life Sci.* **58:** 1929–35.

27 Murata T, Koshino Y, Omori M *et al.* (1993) *In vivo* proton MRS study on premature aging in adult Down's syndrome. *Biol Psychiatry.* **34:** 290–7.

28 Ieshima A, Kisa T, Yoshino K *et al.* (1984) A morphometric CT study of Down's syndrome showing small posterior fossa and calcification of basal ganglia. *Neuroradiology.* **26:** 493–8.

29 Schapiro MB, Creasey H, Schwartz M *et al.* (1987) Quantitative CT analysis of brain morphometry in adult Down's syndrome at different ages. *Neurology.* **37:** 1424–7.

30 Pearlson GD, Warren AC, Starkstein SE *et al.* (1990) Brain atrophy in 18 patients with Down syndrome: a CT study. *Am J Neuroradiol.* **11:** 811–16.

31 Schapiro MB, Luxenberg JS, Kaye JA *et al.* (1989) Serial quantitative CT analysis of brain morphometrics in adult Down's syndrome at different ages. *Neurology.* **39:** 1349–53.

32 Ikeda M and Arai Y (2002) Longitudinal changes in brain CT scans and development of dementia in Down's syndrome. *Eur Neurol.* **47:** 205–8.

33 Maruyama K, Ikeda S and Yanagisawa N (1995) Correlative study of the brain CT and clinical features of patients with Down's syndrome in three clinical stages of Alzheimer-type dementia. *Rinsho Shinkeigaku.* **35:** 775–80.

34 LeMay M, Stafford JL, Sandor T *et al.* (1986) A statistical assessment of perceptual CT scan ratings in patients with Alzheimer-type dementia. *J Comput Assist Tomogr.* **10:** 802–9.

35 Weis S, Weber G, Neuhold A *et al.* (1991) Down syndrome: MR quantification of brain structures and comparison with healthy control subjects. *Am J Neuroradiol.* **12:** 1207–11.

36 Kesslak JP, Nagata BS, Lott I *et al.* (1994) MRI analysis of age-related changes in the brains of individuals with DS. *Neurology.* **44:** 1039–45.

37 Krasuski JS, Alexander GE, Horowitz B *et al.* (2002) Relation of medial temporal volumes to age and memory function in non-demented adults with Down's syndrome: implications for the prodromal phase of Alzheimer's disease. *Am J Psychiatry.* **159:** 74–81.

38 Raz N, Torres IJ, Briggs SD *et al.* (1995) Selective neuroanatomical abnormalities in Down's syndrome and their cognitive correlates: evidence from MRI morphometry. *Neurology.* **45:** 356–66.

39 Aylward EH, Li Q, Habbak QR *et al.* (1997) Basal ganglia volume in adults with Down syndrome. *Psychiatry Res.* **16:** 73–82.

40 Aylward EH, Li Q, Honeycutt NA *et al.* (1999) MRI volumes of the hippocampus and amygdala in adults with Down's syndrome with and without dementia. *Am J Psychiatry.* **156:** 564–8.

41 Pinter JD, Eliez S, Schmitt JE *et al.* (2001) Neuroanatomy of Down's syndrome: a high-resolution MRI study. *Am J Psychiatry.* **158:** 1659–65.

42 Pearlson GD, Breiter SN, Aylward EH *et al.* (1998) MRI brain changes in subjects with Down syndrome with and without dementia. *Dev Med Child Neurol.* **40:** 326–34.

43 White NS, Alkire MT and Haier RJ (2003) A voxel-based morphometric study of non-demented adults with Down syndrome. *Neuroimaging.* **20:** 393–403.

44 Pinter JD, Eliez S, Schmitt JE *et al.* (2001) Amygdala and hippocampal volumes in children with Down syndrome: a high-resolution MRI study. *Neurology.* **56:** 972–4.

45 Jernigan TL and Bellugi U (1990) Anomalous brain morphology on magnetic resonance images in Williams' syndrome and Down syndrome. *Arch Neurol.* **47:** 529–33.

46 Wang PP, Doherty S, Hesselink JR *et al.* (1992) Callosal morphology concurs with neurobehavioral and neuropathological findings in two neurodevelopmental disorders. *Arch Neurol.* **49:** 407–11.

47 Hessl D, Rivera SM and Reiss AL (2004) The neuroanatomy and neuroendocrinology of fragile X syndrome. *Ment Retard Dev Disabil Res Rev.* **10:** 17–24.

48 Schumann CM, Hamstra J, Goodlin-Jones BL *et al.* (2004) The amygdala is enlarged in children but not adolescents with autism; the hippocampus is enlarged at all ages. *J Neurosci.* **24:** 6392–401.

49 Squire LR, Stark CE and Clark RE (2004) The medial temporal lobe. *Annu Rev Neurosci.* **27:** 279–306.

50 Pennington BF, Moon J, Edgin J *et al.* (2003) The neuropsychology of Down syndrome: evidence for hippocampal dysfunction. *Child Dev.* **74:** 75–93.

51 Jernigan TL, Bellugi U, Sowell E *et al.* (1993) Cerebral morphologic distinctions between Williams' and Down syndromes. *Arch Neurol.* **50:** 186–91.

52 Frith U and Frith CD (1974) Specific motor disabilities in Down's syndrome. *J Child Psychol Psychiatry.* **15:** 293–301.

53 Leiner HC, Leiner AL and Dow RS (1993) Cognitive and language functions of the human cerebellum. *Trends Neurosci.* **16:** 444–7.

54 Grafman J, Litvan I, Massaquoi S *et al.* (1992) Cognitive planning deficit in patients with cerebellar atrophy. *Neurology.* **42:** 1493–6.

55 Bracke-Tolkmitt R (1989) The cerebellum contributes to mental skills. *Behav Neurosci.* **103:** 442–6.

56 Ivry RB and Baldo JV (1992) Is the cerebellum involved in learning and cognition? *Curr Opin Neurobiol.* **2:** 212–16.

57 Appollonio IM, Grafman J, Schwartz V *et al.* (1993) Memory in patients with cerebellar degeneration. *Neurology.* **43:** 1536–44.

58 Wang PP (1996) A neuropsychological profile of Down syndrome: cognitive skills and brain morphology. *Ment Retard Dev Disabil Res Rev.* **2:** 102–8.

59 Morrish PK, Sawle GV and Brooks DJ (1996) Regional changes in [^{18}F]dopa metabolism in the striatum in Parkinson's disease. *Brain.* **119:** 2097–103.

60 Teipel SJ, Schapiro MB, Alexander GE *et al.* (2003) Relation of corpus callosum and hippocampal size to age in nondemented adults with Down's syndrome. *Am J Psychiatry.* **160:** 1870–8.

61 Hampel H, Teipel SJ, Alexander GE *et al.* (2002) *In vivo* imaging of region and cell type specific neocortical neurodegeneration in Alzheimer's disease. Perspectives of MRI-

derived corpus callosum measurement for mapping disease progression and effects of therapy. Evidence from studies with MRI, EEG and PET. *J Neural Transm.* **109:** 837–55.

62 Teipel SJ, Alexander GE, Schapiro MB *et al.* (2004) Age-related cortical grey matter reductions in non-demented Down's syndrome adults determined by MRI with voxel-based morphometry. *Brain.* **127:** 811–24.

63 Prasher V, Cumella S, Natarajan K *et al.* (2002) Magnetic resonance imaging, Down's syndrome and Alzheimer's disease: research and clinical implications. *J Intellect Disabil Res.* **46:** 90–100.

Chapter 10

Concluding remarks

Vee P Prasher

Alzheimer's disease (AD) is the commonest form of dementia in older adults with intellectual disability (ID), being particularly associated with Down syndrome (DS). It is estimated that the number of adults with DS who will develop dementia in Alzheimer's disease (DAD) will dramatically increase in the near future. Survival after the onset of the disease is (on average) 6 to 8 years.

In the early twentieth century, our understanding of the lives of people with DS was very much based on a 'medical' approach, textbooks of that time focusing mainly on the physical characteristics of the syndrome. In the mid- to late twentieth century the philosophy of 'community care' became prominent, leading to a more 'social' model of care for people with DS. At the start of the twenty-first century there appears to be a resurgence of interest in the more medical aspects of people with DS. This relates in particular to the biological and genetic aspects of DS, no more so than in the associated condition of AD. Although our knowledge and understanding of AD and DAD in people with DS lag behind that for the general population, as a result of rapid developments in molecular genetics and improvement in neuropathological assessments our understanding of the biological aspects of AD in adults with DS is improving dramatically. Undoubtedly with better understanding of the biopathogenesis of AD, the prevention or cure of DAD in adults with DS will be possible.

There remain concerns about the accurate diagnosis of DAD in people with ID by neuropsychological means alone. As in the general population, the diagnosis of DAD is mainly obtained by excluding other health disorders which may present as dementia. The diagnostic tests and criteria that are available for the general population are often not applicable to people with ID. Neuropsychological testing in older adults with DS often cannot discriminate between 'normal ageing', mild cognitive impairment and DAD.

Although blood tests and brain imaging are routine assessments in adults with possible DAD in the general population and can aid the diagnosis, in the field of ID these investigations are often not undertaken. The development of a highly sensitive and reliable biological marker for DAD in all adults would be a significant advance in medical science. Such a biological marker would need to reflect the neuropathological and neurophysiological mechanisms of AD. It may be that a combination of biological markers will be necessary.

A number of investigatory techniques are now readily accessible (including MRI and CT brain scanning), but no test has yet been established as diagnostic for DAD. At present such investigations at best support the clinical diagnosis of DAD. Often these tests cannot in themselves discriminate between DAD and other types of dementia which may occur in people with ID. Furthermore, such tests still need to develop parameters to differentiate between healthy normal ageing adults with ID and those individuals who have a disease process. It is to be expected that, once limitations of resolution, practicalities and access have been overcome, functional imaging will play a greater role in the assessment and management of DAD in people with ID. Further research is needed to determine whether peripheral blood markers such as beta-amyloid measurements or measurements of the mean corpuscular volume of red blood cells are suitable.

It is probable that the underlying neurochemical, biochemical and neuropathological processes of AD begin many years, if not many decades, before the clinical symptoms of DAD become apparent. Therefore the pathology that is present at the time of the clinical presentation may be the 'end process' to many other processes. At present little research is being undertaken to investigate biological markers for AD in the presymptomatic stage. However, it remains important (for example, to enable appropriate drug intervention for DAD) to improve our understanding of the underlying biological markers that may identify or characterise the disease process before clinical symptomatology appears.

A better understanding of the biological aspects of AD will improve the longevity of people with DS and will also improve the quality of life for this vulnerable population. DAD is and remains the most formidable medical disorder for older adults with ID. Further research into biological aspects is necessary and must continue alongside developments in treatment, and improved community provision.

Index